Meeting the Needs

of

People with Vision Loss

A Multidisciplinary Perspective

Susan L. Greenblatt, Editor

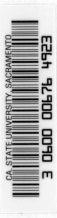
Resources for Rehabilitation
Lexington, Massachusetts

Resources for Rehabilitation
33 Bedford Street, Suite 19A
Lexington, Massachusetts 02173

ISBN 0-929718-07-0

Resources for Rehabilitation is a nonprofit organization dedicated to providing training and information to professionals and the public about the needs of individuals with disabilities and the resources available to meet those needs.

Library of Congress Cataloguing-in-Publication Data
Meeting the Needs of People with Vision Loss: A Multidisciplinary Perspective / Susan L. Greenblatt, editor
   p.   cm.
Includes bibliographical references.
ISBN 0-929718-07-0
1. Blind--Rehabilitation 2. Blind--Services for 3. Low vision
4. Aged, Blind I. Greenblatt, Susan L. II. Resources for Rehabilitation
(Organization)
RA645.B54M44 1991
362.4'1--dc20   91-32812
                                                 CIP

Table of Contents

Multidisciplinary Case Studies

About the Authors

Martha Bagley, M.S., is Specialist to Older Adults at the Helen Keller National Center for Deaf-Blind Youths and Adults at the Dallas Regional Office. Ms Bagley coordinates professional training, provides consultation and technical assistance, and advocates for older adults with vision and hearing impairmẽnts.

Susan Becker, M.Ed., has worked as a social worker with children, a trainer of rehabilitation professionals, and is currently supervisor of an interagency Client Assistance Program at the Massachusetts Commission for the Blind, Boston, Massachusetts.

Monica Beliveau-Tobey, M.Ed., is on the faculty of the Pennsylvania College of Optometry, where she is principal investigator of a federally funded grant that is developing a curriculum on vision and aging for nursing home personnel. She has served as director of a vision impairment program at a nursing home and as consultant to many multidisciplinary projects related to vision and aging.

Marla Bernbaum, M.D., is an Assistant Professor of Internal Medicine at St. Louis University School of Medicine in the Division of Endocrinology. Her primary interest is in the treatment of diabetes and associated complications. She currently directs St. Louis University's diabetes patient education program, which also offers special services to visually impaired patients.

Michael Bina, Ed.D., is Superintendent of the Indiana School for the Blind, Indianapolis, Indiana. He is the President-Elect of the Association for Education and Rehabilitation of the Blind and Visually Impaired, International. He has published articles on such topics as teacher morale, legal liability in orientation and mobility, rural area service delivery, and physical fitness for individuals who are blind or visually impaired.

Barbara Davis, M.Ed., is Director of Rehabilitation and Training at VISION Foundation, Inc. in Watertown, Massachusetts. She is also Lecturer/Clinical Supervisor in the Vision Studies Department at Boston College.

1

Maureen A. Duffy, M.S., is on the faculty of the Department of Graduate Studies in Vision Impairment at Pennsylvania College of Optometry. She has lectured widely on aging and vision loss and has served as a consultant to several agencies.

Lawrence S. Evans, M.D., Ph.D., is Assistant Professor of Ophthalmology at Loyola University Stritch School of Medicine. He has run the Low Vision Service at Loyola since 1979.

Susan L. Greenblatt, Ph.D., is Training Director at Resources for Rehabilitation and Senior Research Sociologist at the Institute for Scientific Research, where she has conducted studies in the areas of education, medicine, and rehabilitation. Her publications have appeared in social science, medical, and rehabilitation journals.

Alice G. Karpik, M.D., is an ophthalmologist in private practice at the Hammond Clinic, Munster, Indiana where she also provides low vision services.

John Mascia, M.A., is Coordinator of Audiological Services at the Helen Keller National Center for Deaf-Blind Youths and Adults in Sands Point, New York. He also is a consulting audiologist for a private practice.

Stanley F. Wainapel, M.D., M.P.H., is Associate Director of the Department of Rehabilitation Medicine at St. Luke's/Roosevelt Hospital Center and Associate Professor of Clinical Rehabilitation at the College of Physicians and Surgeons, Columbia University.

James Warnke, A.C.S.W., is a psychotherapist in private practice in Teaneck, New Jersey and a clinical consultant to the Adjustment to Blindness Project in Denville, New Jersey. He has lectured widely on the issues of psychological adjustment to blindness and visual impairment.

Fran A. Weisse, L.C.S.W., is Resources Director at Resources for Rehabilitation in Lexington, Massachusetts and Information Center Manager at VISION Foundation, Inc. in Watertown, Massachusetts. She has written numerous publications for professional service providers and for people with vision loss. Ms Weisse has worked in the field of blindness rehabilitation for 21 years.

Introduction

Susan L. Greenblatt, Ph.D.

Specialization within the field of medicine, educational develop-
ments within the field of rehabilitation, and technological advances have
all led to an increase in the number and types of professionals who
provide services to individuals with vision loss. This progress naturally
leads to the expectation that individuals with vision loss (or other
disabilities) will benefit from enhanced services. Recent research
(Greenblatt: 1988a,b) has shown that all too often this is not the case.
Instead of enhancing the opportunities for these individuals, fragmentation
among the various specialties often results in a gap in services for people
with vision loss.

The biographical information about the authors of the chapters in this
book reveals the many different professionals who must work together to
achieve the goal of enhanced services. Included are ophthalmologists,
rehabilitation counselors, rehabilitation teachers, an endocrinologist, a
physiatrist, social workers, special educators, an aging specialist, and an
audiologist. Many other professionals play important roles in the process
of helping people with vision loss, including orientation and mobility
instructors, optometrists, occupational and physical therapists, family
physicians, psychologists, and nurses. This volume is an effort to
increase the interdisciplinary communication that is necessary to provide
appropriate services to meet the many needs of people with vision loss.

"What People with Vision Loss Need to Know" reports the results
of interviews conducted with individuals who had experienced vision loss
in the four years prior to the research study. The study asked respon-

*Susan L. Greenblatt, (ed.) Meeting the Needs of People with Vision Loss:
A Multidisciplinary Perspective, Lexington, MA: Resources for
Rehabilitation*

dents about their experiences with a variety of professionals and services, starting with the diagnosis of irreversible vision loss through the receipt of rehabilitation services.

In "Information and Referral Services for People with Vision Loss," Fran A. Weisse discusses the important role these services play in meeting the needs of people with vision loss, how professionals may use existing services, and how they can organize information and referral services in their own practices.

Individuals exist in a social environment; the types of social support systems they have play a major role in determining their responses to vision loss and other disabilities. For most individuals, the family is the foremost source of support. In "The Role of the Family in the Adjustment to Blindness or Visual Impairment," James W. Warnke discusses both healthy and pathological family structures and how they affect the family member who has experienced vision loss. His perceptive analysis will enable service providers to understand why certain individuals have difficulty adjusting, while others manage to cope after going through a period of mourning.

In "Diabetes and Vision Loss: Special Considerations," Marla Bernbaum discusses the variety of health problems that are precipitated by diabetes and how they affect the rehabilitation of individuals whose vision loss is caused by this disease. The psychosocial aspects of diabetes and vision loss and specially adapted equipment that helps individuals who are visually impaired or blind to manage their diabetes are described. Bernbaum also presents the components of a special program that she and her colleagues developed for individuals who are diabetic and visually impaired or blind.

Children and adolescents who are visually impaired or blind live and learn within different institutional structures than adults. All children are subject to peer pressure; must adhere to the requirements of school; and are in the process of developing their own self-identity. Visual impairment or blindness adds an extra dimension to growing up. James W. Warnke, in his chapter, "Special Needs of Children and Adolescents," discusses the stress imposed by visual impairment or blindness, how to adapt activities that are crucial to socialization, how to encourage children

4

and adolescents to use adaptive aids, and the importance of role models who are visually impaired or blind.

"Older Adults with Vision and Hearing Losses," by Martha Bagley, addresses a topic that is too often neglected. Although they are often undetected or misdiagnosed as dementia, dual sensory losses are common among the oldest members of our population. The need for multidisciplinary services is especially important for these individuals. Bagley's chapter discusses how the various medical professionals, rehabilitation professionals, and professionals in the field of aging must develop collaborations and model programs in order to serve this growing population. Although the chapter focuses on older adults with dual sensory losses, the many important points made in the chapter apply to older adults with one sensory loss as well.

"Providing Services to Visually Impaired Elders in Long Term Care Facilities: A Multidisciplinary Approach," by Maureen A. Duffy and Monica Beliveau-Tobey, discusses the prevalence of vision loss among institutionalized elders. The chapter presents an innovative program designed to train staff in these facilities to recognize vision problems and to work with members of other disciplines so that residents are able to function at their maximum level of ability.

A series of case studies follow, written by service providers who represent different disciplines. Readers are advised to analyze each case, keeping in mind the suggestions made in the earlier chapters of the book. Some important issues to consider are:

• Have all the necessary professionals been brought into the case? Do the professionals have adequate communication with each other? Do they provide each other with sufficient information about the patient/client/student, including medical conditions and current visual function? Do they avoid using technical language that is specific to their own discipline? Does each professional provide follow-up information to the other? Has someone taken the responsibility of being case manager? Have the professionals suggested specific mechanisms for increasing multidisciplinary provision of care, i.e., meetings, conference calls, etc.?

• Has enough information been provided to the patient/client/student regarding his or her physical condition, the functional implications, and the services and equipment that can help?

• Has the patient/client/student been given an opportunity to participate in the decision-making process regarding his or her own rehabilitation? In the cases involving children, have parents, school personnel, and the child jointly discussed the case with rehabilitation and medical professionals as well as special educators?

• Was the individual's specific situation, including family life, occupational status, and psychological status, taken into account when deciding a course of action?

Each of the authors of these case studies has worked to provide optimal services to their patients/clients/students. Despite the best efforts of these individual professionals, training programs still fail to educate their students to interact regularly with members of other disciplines. Institutionalized structures to facilitate these interactions are lacking in most settings. This book, along with its companion volume, *Providing Services for People with Vision Loss: A Multidisciplinary Perspective,* was written to stimulate increased attention to a multidisciplinary approach to meeting the needs of people with vision loss and to help establish educational programs and institutionalized structures to meet this goal.

References

Greenblatt, Susan L.
1988a "Physicians and Chronic Impairment: A Study of Ophthalmologists' Interactions with Visually Impaired and Blind Patients" *Social Science and Medicine* 26:4:393-399
1988b "Teaching Ophthalmology Residents about Rehabilitation" *Ophthalmology* 95(October):10:1468-1472

What People with Vision Loss Need to Know*

Susan L. Greenblatt, Ph.D.

What happens to individuals who have learned that there is no medical treatment to restore vision that they have lost? Ideally, such individuals are referred for and receive rehabilitation services that enable them to continue functioning in their daily activities. A recent study (Greenblatt: 1988a) suggests that the ideal pattern of referral from ophthalmologist to rehabilitation agencies may not be the norm. Ophthalmologists receive little training about rehabilitation services, and rehabilitation agencies do not regularly inform ophthalmologists about the services they provide.

Ophthalmologists' own reports about their referrals provide the data for the study referenced above. Unfortunately, current data from either rehabilitation agencies or from individuals who have experienced vision loss are not available. Two major studies conducted in the late 1960's, however, suggest that many people who have experienced vision loss do not receive appropriate services from rehabilitation agencies.

This article reports the findings of interviews conducted with individuals in Massachusetts who had recently experienced vision loss. The purpose of the study was to learn the types of information these individuals received from ophthalmologists and rehabilitation professionals and the types of referrals and services they received.

Previous Research

In the late 1960's, two major studies of the rehabilitation services for individuals who were visually impaired or blind (OSTI:1968; Scott: 1967,1969a,b) were conducted. These studies portrayed a rehabilitation system that did not respond to the changing demographic characteristics

Susan L. Greenblatt, (ed.) Meeting the Needs of People with Vision Loss: A Multidisciplinary Perspective, Lexington, MA: Resources for Rehabilitation

of the visually impaired or blind population; that held rigid stereotypes of the behavior considered appropriate for individuals who were visually impaired or blind; that had few professionally trained employees; and that could be termed a "system" only in the very loosest sense.

Perhaps the finding of greatest importance from these earlier studies is that relatively small proportions of the visually impaired and blind population received services from rehabilitation agencies. The OSTI report (1968) estimated that only about 20% of the blind population received rehabilitation services (excluding income maintenance) and that very few services were available for the "aged blind," even though the aged constituted the largest proportion of the visually impaired or blind population. Those in urban centers were far more likely to receive services than those who lived in rural areas. Scott's (1969a) study reached a similar conclusion, stating that agencies for the blind served what he called the "elite," children and employable adults. Those with the greatest need for services, such as the multiply handicapped, were the least likely to receive rehabilitation services.

Both Scott (1969a) and the OSTI report (1968) concluded that rehabilitation services available at the time were oriented toward totally blind individuals and failed to adapt to the needs of those with residual vision. Scott indicated that a majority of the legally blind population had an acuity at or near the 20/200 level, but the rigidity of the blindness agencies resulted in treating all clients as if they were totally blind. Thus, for example, individuals who would have been capable of reading with magnifiers or other low vision aids were told by agency personnel that they should learn braille. This stereotypical image held by rehabilitation professionals worked to mold individuals who were visually impaired or blind into a behavior pattern of dependence, especially with regard to the agency itself. Scott concluded that even though most agencies indicated that they supported a restorative approach to rehabilitation, that is restoring individuals to an independent lifestyle, in fact most agencies practiced an accommodative approach, or one that works to make blind clients dependent upon the agency.

Despite the numerous findings that portrayed an unresponsive rehabilitation system, the OSTI report did recognize that forces for change were beginning to appear. For example, the supply of the "right" type of client (i.e., employable adults and children with visual impairment as their only disability) was beginning to shrink, suggesting that the rehabilitation agencies would have to begin providing services to the more difficult cases if they were to survive. A change of outlook from vocational rehabilitation to a wider range of services was beginning to surface.

In the two decades that have passed since these studies were carried out, numerous changes have taken place in the field, including the development of technological aids that make independence a more viable goal for individuals who are visually impaired or blind; the expansion of professional training programs for rehabilitation personnel; and the results of the earlier research studies. Indeed, some evidence does exist to indicate that the changes have occurred in the rehabilitation system over the past two decades in response to the critical findings of the studies cited. For example, a survey of rehabilitation agencies listed in the *AFB Directory of Agencies Serving the Visually Handicapped in the U.S.* (Kirchner and Aiello: 1980) found that a wide range of services is provided by a large proportion of agencies. Nearly all of the agencies surveyed provided counseling, training in activities of daily living, and orientation and mobility training. About half of the agencies also provided technological aids that contribute to the independence of individuals who are visually impaired or blind.

Methods

This study was carried out in Massachusetts because the state law requiring that ophthalmologists and optometrists register individuals who are legally blind with the state commission for the blind is the most stringent in the country. Massachusetts is the only state that has a law stipulating a fine for ophthalmologists or optometrists who fail to register individuals who are legally blind. The existence of this law suggests that the register of individuals who are legally blind is the most complete of any in the country. Therefore, the Massachusetts register should offer the opportunity for obtaining the most representative sample of the legally blind population.

The study utilized a variety of methods in order to contact individuals who had experienced vision loss in the four years prior to the research. The Massachusetts Commission for the Blind (MCB) cooperated with the research staff by drawing a sample of individuals who had been registered with the agency during this period. Because of confidentiality requirements imposed by state law, only MCB staff members (not the research project staff) could draw a systematic sample and mail out letters describing the study to sample members. The letter, typed in large print and signed by the Commissioner, requested that the recipients participate in the study and respond by either returning a postage-paid postcard or phoning the principal investigator's office. Recipients were assured that the interviews would be strictly confidential and were informed that they would receive ten dollars for their participation. The principal investigator did not receive a list of names of the entire sample, nor did MCB learn which sample members agreed to participate in the study.

MCB mailed letters to 600 individuals who had been registered initially during the years 1984 through 1987. Of these, 494 actually received the mailing. The other letters were returned because of incorrect addresses or because the individuals were deceased. Eighty individuals responded either by phone or by postcard. Each of these respondents received a phone call from the research staff, during which further explanation of the project was provided; basic demographic data were obtained; and, for those individuals who wished to participate, an appointment for an interview was set up. Some respondents were unable to participate because of physical illness or plans to be away for lengthy periods; others began the interview process and were unable to complete it or were unable to give coherent responses; and others decided against participating before the interview began. A total of 38 usable interviews were obtained from those who responded to the Commissioner's letter.

MCB serves only those individuals who are legally blind. Therefore, other methods were used to reach individuals who are visually impaired but not legally blind and individuals who are legally blind but not registered with the MCB. Announcements describing the study were sent to every private agency in the state that serves individuals who are visually impaired or blind. The principal investigator requested that these agencies publicize the study over telephone information tapes, in newsletters, and at meetings. In addition, the radio reading services made regular announcements about the study.

Fifty-five individuals responded to the announcements made by private agencies. However, many of these individuals were congenitally blind and had not been initially registered during the 1984 to 1987 study period; therefore, they were not eligible to participate in the study. Ten usable interviews were obtained from these sources.

An analysis of the response patterns raises an important but often neglected issue. Individuals who are visually impaired but not legally blind, although they constitute the largest proportion of the visually impaired population (Greenblatt: 1988b), were very difficult to locate. Despite the variety of methods used to recruit these individuals throughout the state, only three individuals who are visually impaired but not legally blind responded. This suggests that people who are not legally blind have very little knowledge of or access to services. In fact, the few respondents in this category of visual impairment stressed the difficulty that they had had in locating services. These individuals only managed to find services through serendipitous means. For example, in one case a man read an announcement about self-help groups for people with vision loss in a local newspaper and mentioned the notice to his wife, who had recently experienced vision loss. She was able to walk from her home to the meeting site, where she found a group of people who were in situations similar to her own.

Several factors suggest that the respondents may not constitute a representative sample. Although MCB conducts an annual census requesting changes of address, the relatively high rate of returned mail suggests that the register is not as accurate as it could be. The high percentage of incorrect addresses may introduce a bias into the sample, as individuals who fail to respond to MCB's annual census may have a different perception of the agency than those who complete the annual census. In addition, the fact that some individuals were unable to participate because of other health problems or disabilities introduces an additional bias and makes it difficult to obtain information about serving individuals with multiple disabilities. Furthermore, the difficulty in obtaining responses from individuals who are not legally blind introduces yet another bias into the study. Despite these possible statistical biases, the information provided by the respondents presented such clear patterns that the research staff was convinced that the findings provide important insights for professionals who work with people with vision loss.

Findings

The interviews were designed to elicit information about how the respondents discovered that their vision loss was irreversible; the information they received from ophthalmologists and other service providers; and the types of rehabilitation services they received. Respondents were asked when and how they were referred for rehabilitation; if they were referred to more than one agency; and the types of agencies that provided services.

Four-fifths of the respondents (81.3%) were females and over three-fifths (61.7%) were over age 65. The most frequent cause of visual impairment or blindness in the sample (see Table 1) was macular degeneration (31.9%), followed by diabetic retinopathy (21.3%). At the time the vision loss first occurred, about a third of the respondents (32.6%) were retired, another third (30.4%) were employed, and just over a fifth (21.7%) were homemakers (see Table 2). Most of the respondents (85.7%) had been referred to MCB by their ophthalmologist.

The first set of questions concerned what the ophthalmologists told the respondents about their visual status, about legal blindness, and about rehabilitation services. Although most ophthalmologists (81.1%) told patients they would be registered with MCB, only about a quarter of the respondents (24.3%) received explanations about legal blindness from their ophthalmologists. Nor did the ophthalmologists describe the services MCB offered. The impact of the term legal blindness had serious effects on some of the respondents, but when they received an accurate definition of the term and realized it was not a medical prognosis, their anxieties were alleviated. For example, one respondent indicated that legal blindness did not mean anything to her because, "I already knew that I couldn't see and I was in trouble."

Table 1   **Cause of vision loss**

	%
Macular degeneration	31.9
Diabetic retinopathy	21.3
Retinitis pigmentosa	6.4
Glaucoma	6.4
Cataracts	6.4
Retinopathy of prematurity	4.3
Albinism	2.1
Other	21.3

Table 2   **Primary activity at time of vision loss**

Retired	32.6
Employed	30.4
Homemaker	21.7
Student	2.2
Other	13.0

Table 3   **Respondents who received:**

Talking books	77.8
Orientation and mobility	46.8
Rehabilitation teaching	46.3

Table 4   **Respondents who had used:**

Magnifiers/optical aids	81.8
Cane or guide dog	57.8
Large print books	43.2
Volunteers for shopping/reading	20.0
Radio reading services	15.6
Telephone tapes at agencies	11.1
Closed circuit televisions	9.1
Adapted computer equipment	2.2

Prior to their own experiences with MCB, less than a third of the respondents (28.6%) had known about MCB or the services it offers to help individuals cope with vision loss. Although all but one of the legally blind respondents received at least one visit from a staff member from MCB, the type of information and services that respondents received varied greatly (see Table 3). The most consistently offered service was talking books, provided to over three-quarters of the respondents (77.8%). Just under half of the respondents (48.8%) received orientation and mobility instruction (with some receiving only one lesson), and a similar proportion (46.3%) received rehabilitation teaching, usually in the form of marking appliances throughout the home. Of the 14 individuals who had been employed when their vision loss first occurred, only one was told about vocational counseling and received this service. In contrast to the findings of the earlier studies, a minority of the respondents received financial benefits from MCB; only a fifth received medical assistance (21.4%) and a similar proportion (19.0%) received supplemental security income.

Many respondents were unaware of a variety of aids and devices or services that could have helped to improve their lifestyle (see Table 4). Of the aids and devices or services listed, the most frequently used were magnifiers/optical aids and canes. The least frequently used were adapted computer equipment, closed circuit televisions, and telephone tapes at agencies.

Referrals by a staff member from MCB to other agencies were made for nearly two-fifths (38.1%) of the respondents. In a few instances, these referrals were made to a comprehensive residential rehabilitation program, while in other instances they were made to low vision specialists or to a private service agency. Few referrals were made by ophthalmologists, optometrists, social workers, or other service providers. Only five respondents (10.4%) indicated that their ophthalmologist had referred them for any services other than those provided by MCB. One might conclude that the ophthalmologists felt that MCB's services were sufficient; however, few respondents indicated that their ophthalmologist told them anything about MCB's services, suggesting that the ophthalmologists themselves probably were not familiar with MCB's services. Less than a third of the respondents (31.9%) contacted agencies on their own, because they were unaware that services existed.

Since few services, referrals, or adaptive aids were provided to the respondents, what did happen when rehabilitation professionals visited the respondents' homes? It was common for rehabilitation professionals to tell the respondents, "Call if you need anything." But the respondents did not know what services were available, so they were unable to say what they needed. A poignant example of this phenomenon involved an older woman who had both macular degeneration and detached retinas. This woman was afraid of falling inside her home and did not go outside on her own. When asked if she had told the rehabilitation professional about this problem, she responded, "What good would it do? Nothing can be done about it." Had this woman known about orientation and mobility training and in fact received it, her life could have changed significantly.

Conclusions and Recommendations

The majority of respondents are individuals who would like services but, because they are unknowledgeable about the services that exist, are unable to obtain them. Some individuals do not understand that they are entitled to services, while others think that they are too old to receive services.

Those respondents who are younger and more assertive by nature are more likely to persist in efforts to obtain information and services. These individuals aggressively seek all possible services. They learn to work the system and are persistent. As one young woman said about rehabilitation professionals:

> They're elusive. They don't tell the whole story of what
> is available. Getting the information is like pulling teeth.
> People need a stubborn streak to seek out information
> because of the lack of information provided.

Those who moved into the state during the study period and who already knew what services were available (usually those who were congenitally blind and had grown up with these services) knew just what services and aids to ask for and received them promptly. For example, a man who worked for the Internal Revenue Service told the staff of MCB that he needed orientation and mobility training in the areas around his new home and his place of employment. He also requested adaptive equipment with speech output. His requests were filled promptly, because he was able to state exactly what he needed.

A few respondents received referrals from other health professionals and received services that enabled them to remain independent. One young woman, a nurse who became totally blind due to diabetic retinopathy, sought medical treatment in several prestigious institutions. Although the ophthalmologists who examined her all failed to tell her about rehabilitation services, her diabetologist did refer her to a residential rehabilitation center, where she learned how to live independently. Upon completion of this program, the woman began living on her own and had plans to marry.

Some respondents never completely accepted their vision loss and continued to be hostile to professional service providers. One respondent who had diabetic retinopathy but was not legally blind believed that no services were appropriate for her. During the interview, this respondent said:

> Ophthalmologists don't talk about the progression of the disease... They are very careful not to talk about the future. They don't want you to be depressed.

This respondent was angry not only at her ophthalmologist but also at rehabilitation agencies, which she thought were "unreal" in their expectations of what their clients could achieve. For this respondent, therapy with a counselor who specialized in grief and loss was the only service that was helpful. Other individuals who did not accept the permanence of vision loss, even after years, made statements such as, "I'm not blind really" or "I hope I'll grow out of it."

A few respondents were dissatisfied with the services they received and complained to staff members at MCB as well as to the interviewer. These individuals were usually parents of children who were visually impaired or blind.

Several respondents were extremely dependent on spouses or other family members in order to carry out their daily activities. These individuals often stated that they did not know how they would cope without their spouse. It is likely that these individuals will be institutionalized if the sighted spouse dies before they do.

In sum, many people are unaware of the many services that exist to help individuals with visual impairment or blindness keep functioning. Lack of knowledge about these services may be attributed to inadequate public education as well as fragmentation between the medical and rehabilitation professions. Even after individuals are registered with MCB, they do not receive complete explanations about the available services.

Agencies no longer have an accommodative approach toward their clients as they did at the time of Scott's study (1967; 1969a,b); rather, they place the burden on the client to contact them if they have any additional needs and to learn about available services on their own. Although elders comprised the majority of respondents, they were less likely to receive services than younger individuals. The lack of referrals made by ophthalmologists, rehabilitation professionals, and other service providers suggest that there is fragmentation not only between the health and rehabilitation professions but also among rehabilitation professionals.

The findings suggest that medical and rehabilitation service providers can do much to improve the conditions of people who have experienced vision loss. Individuals are often in shock upon first hearing the diagnosis of irreversible vision loss. In order to ensure that patients understand their diagnosis and the availability of rehabilitation services, ophthalmologists should schedule follow-up appointments during which they encourage patients to ask questions and obtain information. Physicians, although not expected to be psychologists, need to recognize the differences in patients and to provide the type of information amenable to the educational level and emotional status of the patient. Providing appropriate information can help prevent denial of the permanence of vision loss and encourage patients to seek out services. As Weston and Lipkin have stated:

Giving information to patients requires different skills than taking information from patients: being well organized, clear, avoiding jargon, and tailoring the information to what the patient is able to cope with. (1989: p. 54)

There will always be some people who remain angry or fail to accept their vision loss. For these people, ophthalmologists can only offer information and indicate that services are available if they ever decide they want them. At a time when the patient's anxiety level and fear are already high, anticipating a visit from a government employee may cause increased anxiety, unless the patient knows what to expect. But all patients should be told that they are entitled to services and receive a description of those services. Then they can make the decision themselves whether or not to seek out services. Those who are reluctant to accept services may benefit from meeting another patient who has successfully adapted to vision loss.

Rehabilitation professionals should also provide complete information about available services as well as eligibility criteria for services. Telling clients "to call if you need anything" places an undue burden upon people who have never had any experience with the rehabilitation system. After learning that there are no medical options to help them, most individuals experience fear and a sense of helplessness. Placing the burden on them to request specific services reinforces the sense that "nothing more can be done." Providing information about the wide array of services, training programs, and adaptive equipment may encourage individuals to take positive steps toward regaining their independence.

Both ophthalmologists and rehabilitation professionals should encourage the establishment of self-help groups. Ophthalmologists and their staff members may sometimes overhear the beginnings of a self-help group in the office waiting room. Such sharing of anxieties and solutions to common problems may prove extremely valuable to people who have recently experienced vision loss. In fact, several respondents to this study indicated that talking to others in similar situations was the most valuable help they received, even when they attended formal rehabilitation programs (See Weisse: 1989 for a discussion of how professionals can establish self-help groups for patients or clients.)

In spite of the fact that many respondents to this study had multiple health problems, most rated their health as good. They were coping on their own and were upbeat about their lives. Yet many of the respondents and others who have experienced vision loss could have an improved quality of life if they were provided with accurate and complete information about the wide variety of rehabilitation services available. Provision of this information requires that ophthalmologists and rehabilitation professionals establish ongoing networks of information exchange and disseminate information to patients and to the general public.

References

Greenblatt, Susan L.
1988a "Physicians and Chronic Impairment: A Study of Ophthalmologists' Interactions with Visually Impaired and Blind Patients" *Social Science and Medicine* 26:4:393-399
1988b "Teaching Ophthalmology Residents about Rehabilitation" *Ophthalmology* 95(October):10:1468-1472

Kirchner, Corinne and Robert Aiello
1980 "Services Available to Blind and Visually Handicapped Persons in the U.S.: A Survey of Agencies" *Journal of Visual Impairment and Blindness* 74(June):241-244

Organization for Social and Technical Innovation (OSTI)
1968 *Blindness and Services to the Blind in the U.S. A Report to the Subcommittee on Rehabilitation,* National Institute of Neurological Diseases and Blindness

Scott, Robert A.
1969a *The Making of Blind Men* New York, NY: Russell Sage Foundation
1969b "The System Analysis Approach to Relationships between Agencies for the Blind and Blind Persons" pp. 404-412 in Maxwell H. Goldberg and John R. Swinton (eds.) *Blindness Research: The Expanding Frontier* University Park, PA: Pennsylvania State University Press
1967 "The Selection of Clients by Social Welfare Agencies: The Case of the Blind" *Social Problems* 14(Winter):248-257

Weisse, Fran A,

1989   "Self-Help Groups for People with Vision Loss" pp. 84-99 in
Susan L. Greenblatt (ed.) *Providing Services for People with
Vision Loss: A Multidisciplinary Perspective* Lexington, MA:
Resources for Rehabilitation

Weston, W. Wayne and Mack Lipkin Jr.

1989   "Doctors Learning Communication Skills: Developmental
Issues" pp. 443-57 in Moira Stewart and Debra Roter (eds.)
Communicating with Patients Newbury Park, CA: Sage

* Support for the research reported in this chapter was provided by a
grant awarded to the Institute for Scientific Research by the U.S. Department of Education (H133C80073). Opinions expressed are not necessarily those of the funding agency.

Information and Referral Services for People with Vision Loss

Fran A. Weisse, L.C.S.W.

• *I have been losing my vision for the last three years. I live alone and am afraid that I will be sent to a nursing home if my vision gets worse. Isn't there anything that can be done to help me?*
An 82 year old woman with macular degeneration

• *My three year old daughter had a brain tumor removed and now has bilateral tunnel vision. I am petrified when I think of her future. How will she get through school? How will she live on her own? What if she loses all of her vision?*
A 23 year old mother

• *My sister-in-law has been told that she has macular degeneration and that there is nothing that the doctor can do for her. She has seen three eye doctors and they each say the same thing. What about magnifiers and sunglasses? Where else can she go for care?*
A 67 year old man

The questions posed by these individuals are typical of the many requests for information that I receive in my position as an information and referral (I and R) specialist. During the past 21 years, I have spoken with hundreds, perhaps thousands, of people who did not know where to turn to obtain information that would help them cope with vision loss. Although some of these individuals were referred by health care or rehabilitation professionals, many others found out about the I and R services at VISION Foundation (where I work) by serendipitous conversations with family members, friends, co-workers, or new acquaintances. Often people who contact me have gone months or even years thinking

Susan L. Greenblatt, (ed.) Meeting the Needs of People with Vision Loss: A Multidisciplinary Perspective, Lexington, MA: Resources for Rehabilitation

that there is nothing that can help them live independently with their vision loss. In reality, there is such a vast array of services and products that most people require some direction to find those that are best suited to their needs.

In this chapter, I will describe how to organize an I and R service so that people with vision loss can locate appropriate services and products. The examples are based on my experiences at VISION Foundation, Inc., a support organization for individuals coping with vision loss.

The Need for Information and Referral Services

Several studies provide empirical support for my personal observations that many people leave their ophthalmologists' offices and even rehabilitation agencies without knowing about the many services and products that can help them. For example, Greenblatt (1988) found that many ophthalmologists are unaware of specialized services for people with vision loss, including orientation and mobility training, special services for elders, and special education programs. Obviously, when ophthalmologists are not aware of services, they cannot refer patients who might benefit from them. A study of individuals who had experienced vision loss (see Chapter 1 in this volume) corroborated the findings from the survey of ophthalmologists; most respondents had received very little information about services from their ophthalmologists.

Such findings are not unique to those who work in the field of vision. A recent study regarding provision of information to people with a variety of disabilities found that most of the respondents had received little information from the medical community and had difficulty locating special equipment, financial assistance, and descriptions of available services (Mayfield-Smith: 1990).

While physicians and rehabilitation professionals should expect individuals to go through a period of depression after learning that their vision loss is irreversible, the knowledge that there are services, products, and support groups can help shorten the period of depression and encourage patients with vision loss to continue with their normal activities, with some adaptations and adjustments.

As Kaplan and her colleagues noted:

> It is possible that greater information supplied by the doctor, in the form of instruction, education, or explanation, may contribute to patients' understanding, sense of well-being, and/or confidence regarding the management of their disease. Doctors may in fact influence the outcomes of patients with chronic illness, not only by competent medical care but also by shaping how patients feel about the disease, their sense of commitment to the treatment process, and their ability to control or contain its impact on their lives (1989: p. 244).

As specialization within the health care field has increased, the field of I and R has developed as a specialty in its own right. Although one might argue that adding another specialty results in an increased fragmentation of services to people with medical problems, if used properly I and R services can complement the work of health care and rehabilitation professionals. Indeed, knowing when and how to use I and R services can contribute to a coordinated approach to the provision of services. In fact, many consumers receive more comprehensive information from an I and R specialist who suggests multidisciplinary resources than from a specialist with a narrower perspective.

I and R services provide a vital link between the person with a chronic condition or impairment (in this case, vision loss) and the vast array of services and support groups that are available. Because so many services exist and because they have different eligibility criteria, such as level of visual impairment, age, employment status, and income, it is often necessary for a knowledgeable professional to help the person who has recently been diagnosed with irreversible vision loss to navigate the maze.

In order to prevent individuals with vision loss from falling into the cracks between the health care system and rehabilitation system, health care and rehabilitation professionals alike need to learn more about the role of I and R services. Whether they offer these services themselves or refer individuals with vision loss to I and R networks, professionals should understand that I and R services supplement medical and rehabilitative care. I and R may be appropriate both during and after medical intervention and rehabilitation training, depending upon the specific circumstances of the individual case. I and R provides a self-help aspect to the individual's adjustment to loss of vision. When individuals obtain information that can help them to remain independent, their sense of control over their own lives increases, especially when progressive loss of vision has eroded this sense of control.

Where to Find Information and Referral Services

I and R services may be provided by generic community organizations such as the United Way, often under the umbrella term "First Call" or "First Call for Help." In rural areas where special I and R services for people with vision loss are not available, the United Way I and R service is a good place to seek help.

In both urban and rural communities, the public library is the first source of information about that community's services for individuals in need. The reference librarian often performs the role of the I and R specialist, helping individuals locate directories of community services; suggesting books which describe disabilities and rehabilitation; and recommending other information sources. Many libraries have files of service brochures and bulletin boards where community activities are announced. Some libraries host meetings of organizations and support groups where information and resources are discussed by participants and guest speakers, including the library staff. Some libraries have special access centers which serve individuals with disabilities, and some librarians receive special training in the use of adaptive equipment in order to teach patrons. These access centers and services expand the traditional role of libraries, enabling the person with vision loss to use library materials which were formerly inaccessible.

State rehabilitation services for individuals who are visually impaired or blind may provide I and R services to their clients. Private rehabilitation agencies, independent living centers, consumer organizations, and regional libraries for the blind and physically handicapped may also offer I and R services to individuals with vision loss.

The Components of an I and R Service

Information is provided in many ways and in varying levels of detail. Some individuals request only the name, telephone number, and address of an agency that provides specific services and will do the rest of the work learning about the services and eligibility criteria themselves. Other individuals require detailed information about the service agency, such as eligibility requirements and application procedures. Referral involves the assessment of an inquiry, an evaluation of appropriate resources, and linking the individual with service providers.

I and R specialists must know how to elicit enough information from individuals to make appropriate referrals. In many cases, the initial question is only the first step in what may become a thorough discussion of rehabilitation issues, sources for peer counseling, adaptive aids for employment or daily living, or how to obtain detailed medical information. Many I and R specialists also follow up with the individual to ascertain that the contact has been made. Since many information requests are answered during the course of one telephone conversation, the I and R office must be organized for maximum efficiency, and information must be readily accessible both by topic and geographical location of services.

Some of the basic components of any I and R service are directories, resource files, and educational material for distribution. A new I and R service may simply use an alphabetical list of agencies and organizations. As the service grows, however, subject indexes will quickly become necessary. Rol-a-dex files are very helpful for the I and R service, especially for quick answers to simple inquiries about addresses and telephone numbers. At VISION Foundation, where individuals with vision loss work and receive services, I find that 4 inch by 6 inch Rol-a-dex cards with information in large print are invaluable.

The information may also be written in braille on these cards if it is required by a staff member. The easy removal and replacement of Rol-a-dex cards makes these options possible. Several Rol-a-dex filing systems are useful: an alphabetical Rol-a-dex of organizations frequently contacted; a geographical Rol-a-dex for quick reference to services provided by city; and two Rol-a-dexes which contain entries for the agency's library, one organized by subjects and the other by authors and titles. At VISION Foundation, the I and R Center's computerized database uses the same keywords as the Rol-a-dex system, such as "adaptive aids," "computers and technology," "education," "housing," "rehabilitation," and "transportation."

Computers are especially useful in organizations which employ individuals with vision loss, since computers with large print or speech output make information easily accessible to these individuals. Mayfield-Smith (1990) found that 76% of disability-related I and R systems used computers to provide I and R services, compared to 61.5% of general I and R services. Her study also cited a move toward staffing I and R services with consumers; more than 55% of the I and R services which responded to the study had staff members who had disabilities or who were related to an individual with a disability. Nearly three-quarters of the staff members at I and R services for people with disabilities had disabilities themselves.

The information about organizations included in an I and R center's Rol-a-dex files or computerized database should include address, phone number, hours and days of service, fees and how to pay for services, contact person (s); eligibility requirements (age, income eligibility, etc.); area served; application procedures; lists of specialists/experts; and the date on which the information was entered or updated. Regular updating of information is crucial for a successful I and R service. Recording the month and year of information entry on the Rol-a-dex card or in the computerized database helps to ensure that the information is always current.

I also use a collection of basic reference materials which are kept within arm's reach of my desk and telephone. These materials allow me to answer a telephone question quickly and efficiently. Among these references are a *Dictionary of Visual Science* (Chilton Book Company);

26

adaptive aids catalogues; the *Rehabilitation Resource Manual: VISION,
Living with Low Vision: A Resource Guide for People with Sight Loss,*
and *Resources for Elders with Disabilities,* (Resources for Rehabilitation); community service directories of housing, transportation, mental
health services, special education, and other resources; a road atlas, for
locating the consumer's hometown in order to recommend the nearest
service providers; and a directory of services for individuals with vision
loss in my state. I also use local telephone directories to look up telephone numbers for individuals who cannot read the listings themselves.

Information and referral specialists may need to suggest information about recording techniques, especially when serving individuals who
have recently experienced vision loss. A cassette tape recorder is very
useful to individuals who cannot read written information. Many individuals with vision loss keep a cassette recorder beside their telephones
for taking messages and retrieving information.

Most consumers ask for information on eye diseases, adaptive aids,
financial assistance, local services, hobbies and recreation, and help in
coping with the emotional aspects of vision loss. "Where can I get a
free or low cost eye examination or glasses?" is one of the most common
questions I receive. The VISION Foundation I and R Center developed
an annotated bibliography of "Free or Low Cost Low Vision Services in
Massachusetts" to provide the answers. When I find that an individual
has not been referred for low vision services, I offer to send information
about what to expect from a low vision evaluation and a list of low vision
services in the state. It is often difficult for individuals who have
received a diagnosis of irreversible vision loss to think of all the questions they should ask the doctors. VISION Foundation distributes a
brochure, "Questions to Ask Your Eye Doctor." The list of questions,
developed through the comments of self-help group members, gives
patients guidelines to use during their medical appointment. (Also see
Living with Low Vision: A Resource Guide for People with Sight Loss,
Chapter 1, for a set of relevant questions.)

I and R centers use a variety of staffing options to provide services.
At VISION Foundation, part-time staff and volunteers jointly run the I
and R Center. Normally sighted individuals read the print material to
retrieve and record information for the files and computerized database.

Students from local university internship programs work in the I and R Center. Additional sources of volunteers include optometry schools; professional preparation programs that train teachers and special educators; schools of library science; community colleges; disabled student services; and patients or clients. Low vision service providers, including ophthalmologists, optometrists, and rehabilitation professionals, may also recruit such individuals to provide I and R services in their offices. It is also a good idea for rehabilitation agencies to require that all direct service staff work in the I and R center for several hours each month. This ongoing experience serves to keep staff up-to-date on new resources and adaptive aids.

Many individuals who are visually impaired or blind work as volunteers in each of VISION Foundation's programs. These individuals volunteer in order to develop self-confidence, to learn new skills, and to gain experience which will help them re-enter the job market. An I and R center may also serve as a training program for rehabilitation clients to provide I and R services, as volunteers, on a stipend basis, or as an internship.

Information and referral services are usually provided over the telephone, often with written follow-up; however, it is a good idea to invite consumers who are pursuing information about adaptive aids and rehabilitation services to visit the I and R office, talk with the I and R specialist, and use the library and literature files. Staff or volunteers should demonstrate the adaptive technology they use to perform their work and give the consumer hands-on experience, if possible. When consumers see that they can continue to work independently with adaptive aids, they become more motivated to seek rehabilitation training, and their depression may begin to subside.

A toll-free telephone line encourages maximum use of I and R services. If a national toll-free number is unfeasible, a statewide number is a good alternative. Toll-free numbers which provide access to health and disability services as well as other consumer needs are often listed in the front of telephone directories in sections such as *Community Services Numbers: A Self-Help Guide*.

A very cost-effective and popular supplement to an I and R center's services is a telephone information tape. Many organizations have telephone answering machines for after-hours messages. At VISION Foundation, taped messages recorded twice a week announce events of special interest, information about new adaptive aids and services, legislative alerts, and recreational activities. The answering machine is set up to answer both our local telephone line and our toll-free line, so that anyone in Massachusetts may call without incurring long distance charges. The machine has a counter on it so that we can keep track of the number of calls received.

The basic I and R center for individuals with vision loss described above may be enhanced with:

- a display case of adaptive aids to show to visitors

- a bulletin board with brochures, program announcements, and activities schedules

- LARGE PRINT lists of community agencies and telephone numbers for distribution

- audio and/or video tapes on eye diseases and conditions, rehabilitation techniques, or adaptive equipment, available on loan

- low vision simulators to be used by staff members to help educate family members and others about the functional impact of vision loss

- a special receiver for the local radio reading service

- a Talking Book record player and cassette player for demonstration

- LARGE PRINT reading material in the waiting room or reception area

The I and R center should be a model setting where the physical environment is both safe and readily accessible to people with vision loss. Good lighting, contrasting colors in the interior design, and adaptive equipment for use by staff and clients contribute to the consumer's knowledge and sense of well-being.

I and R services are usually provided without charge to the individual who requests assistance. The expenses of providing I and R services are funded by the host agency through grants from community organizations such as the United Way. In the professional's office, I and R services pay for themselves through word-of-mouth referrals from satisfied "customers."

Ethical Considerations in Providing I and R Services

I and R specialists encounter many ethical considerations in daily service delivery. Individuals frequently request referrals or evaluations of specific ophthalmologists, optometrists, or rehabilitation programs or request a telephone diagnosis of an eye disease or condition. I and R specialists must remain impartial and refrain from endorsing specific health care providers or rehabilitation programs. The I and R specialist should direct consumers to physician referral services or to the local medical, ophthalmology, or optometry society, which in turn will suggest several local practitioners.

Consumers ask I and R specialists questions about eye diseases and conditions when they do not receive this information from their doctors or when they did not understand the information they received. I and R specialists should provide written information obtained from medical sources but should never express personal opinions which lead the consumer to think that the I and R specialist is a medical specialist. I use the reference books and literature sources described earlier in this chapter to develop an information packet to send to consumers. It is also very useful for the I and R specialist to consult with the medical librarian at a nearby medical center, university, or ophthalmology research organization. The medical librarian may perform a literature search for information on both common and unusual eye diseases and conditions. The results of the literature search may be sent to the consumer and added to the agency library for future reference.

When consumers call with complaints about physicians or rehabilitation service providers, the I and R specialist may suggest mediation techniques but should not offer an opinion about a specific individual or agency. Problems may be resolved when the consumer seeks a second medical opinion, contacts the Client Assistance Program of the state office of handicapped affairs, or speaks with a supervisor in a hospital, medical practice, or rehabilitation agency.

Staff members and volunteers must be trained to respect the confidentiality of any individual who requests services. I have found this to be particularly important in an office where staff or volunteers who are visually impaired may not realize that there are others present. Callers' requests and problems must not be discussed where others can overhear. Consultations with other staff members or volunteers often yield solutions to callers' problems; however, the identity of the caller should remain confidential.

Individuals who contact I and R services should be considered "callers" or "consumers" whether they are medical or rehabilitation professionals, parents or adult offspring of individuals with vision loss, or individuals with vision loss themselves. At a self-help organization such as VISION Foundation, individuals must initiate the request for information themselves in order to receive services. Friends or family members may request information for their own use; however, we will not send unsolicited literature or call any individuals who have not contacted us themselves. This self-help requirement may not apply at generic I and R services or in agencies that place less emphasis on self-help.

Many consumers call and express anger or frustration about a diagnosis or prognosis. It is useful to refer these consumers to self-help groups, where they express their concerns to others who have had similar experiences. In many states, self-help groups for adults with vision loss meet to provide emotional support and practical information (see Weisse, "Self-Help Groups for People with Sight Loss," 1989). Where participation in a self-help group is not possible, a telephone reassurance program achieves many of the same goals. In such a program, individuals with vision loss are matched with others who have had similar experiences. Through telephone conversations these "telephone buddies" share information and provide support to one another.

Providing I and R Services in the Professional's Office

Medical and rehabilitation professionals can easily integrate I and R services into their office environment. Patients or clients will benefit from onsite service delivery, especially individuals who lack the self-confidence or motivation to make the initial contact with I and R services on their own.

A staff member should be designated to maintain the files and keep literature up-to-date. This individual should have time in his or her schedule to talk at length with patients or clients to determine their needs and make specific referrals. Although the information in a professional's office may not be as detailed as that in an I and R service, some of the descriptions provided above will help professionals to initiate this service. Minimal requirements of an onsite service are:

- A Rol-a-dex file with the names, addresses, and telephone numbers of qualified, competent rehabilitation agencies, professionals, and counselors who are sensitive to patients' needs and fears.

- LARGE PRINT lists of community agencies which provide services such as transportation, meals-on-wheels, self-help groups, and recreation

- LARGE PRINT literature which describes eye diseases and conditions, rehabilitation services, and adaptive aids, such as those published by Resources for Rehabilitation (see pages 138-140)

Patients or clients who leave the professional's office with this information in hand will have taken the first step toward rehabilitation. In learning about their eye condition and rehabilitation services, they will develop a sense of control over their lives. Information about community services will reduce the fear of isolation often experienced by individuals with vision loss. Brochures and catalogues of adaptive aids will teach them about the devices available to help them maintain their independence.

Professional Resources for the I and R Specialist

I and R specialists need a resource network in order to maintain up-to-date records and receive new information. Books, journals, newsletters, service brochures, product literature, and colleagues provide a constant supply of new information. The Alliance of Information and Referral Systems (AIRS) is a national membership organization for I and R specialists and I and R systems. AIRS chapters in many states offer training programs and workshops to members. The AIRS journal, "Information and Referral," and the "AIRS Newsletter" discuss issues related to the impact of I and R systems on design and delivery of human services. United Way organizations in both the United States and Canada provide I and R services and also offer training programs and resources to local I and R specialists. (Addresses for these organizations are listed at the end of this chapter.) Other professional organizations, research institutions, and references are listed in the *Rehabilitation Resource Manual: VISION* (Resources for Rehabilitation).

Conclusion

Providing information and referral services to individuals with vision loss and to their families not only calms their fears, but also channels their energy into productive activities. Reading about their condition; contacting organizations; talking with peers; and locating adaptive equipment enable people with vision loss to achieve their own individual goals.

The callers cited at the beginning of this chapter all benefited by receiving I and R services:

• The 82 year old woman with macular degeneration was referred to VISION Foundation's Visually Impaired Elders Program for home-based rehabilitation teaching services. This program has taught her to use a microwave oven and a hand-held magnifier to read directions and recipes. Since she has useful peripheral vision, she is comfortable within her own home and moves freely about, now that the edges of her steps have been marked with bright yellow tape. She now acts as a telephone buddy to another woman in similar circumstances; they talk frequently, exchanging news of grandchildren, favorite television programs, and tips about accomplishing everyday activities with vision loss.

• The young mother whose daughter had a brain tumor removed, leaving her with bilateral visual field loss, received an annotated bibliography of "Information Sources for Parents of Children with Vision Loss." This list provided information about support groups, a toll-free information service for parents of toddlers with vision loss, sources of special toys to help her daughter learn to use her remaining vision to the fullest extent possible, and the names of organizations which offer early intervention programs to prepare youngsters with disabilities for school.

• The man who was asking questions on behalf of his sister-in-law received information about macular degeneration, a copy of "Questions To Ask Your Eye Doctor" and information about a national self-help organization for individuals with macular degeneration. He was not given the names of specific physicians but was sent a list of low vision services in the state.

References

Cline, David, Henry W. Hofstetter, and John R. Griffin
1980   *Dictionary of Visual Science* Radnor, PA: Chilton Book Company

Greenblatt, Susan L.
1988   "Physicians and Chronic Impairment: A Study of Ophthalmologists" Interactions with Blind and Visually impaired Patients" *Social Science and Medicine* 26:4:393-399

Kaplan, Sherrie H., Sheldon Greenfield, and John E. Ware, Jr.
1989   "Impact of the Doctor-Patient Relationship on the Outcomes of Chronic Disease" pp. 228-245 in Moira Stewart and Debra Roter (eds.) *Communicating with Medical Patients* New York, NY: Sage Publications

Mayfield-Smith, K.L., G.G. Yajnik, T.L. Toon, and R. Morse
1990   *Study to Determine the Desirability and Feasibility of a Nation-wide Information and Referral System for Persons with Developmental Disabilities: Executive Summary* Columbia, SC: University of South Carolina, Center for Developmental Disabilities

Resources for Rehabilitation
1990   *Living with Low Vision: A Resource Guide for People with Sight Loss* Lexington, MA: Resources for Rehabilitation
1990   *Rehabilitation Resource Manual: VISION* Lexington, MA: Resources for Rehabilitation
1990   *Resources for Elders with Disabilities* Lexington, MA: Resources for Rehabilitation

Weisse, Fran
1989   "Self-Help Groups for People with Sight Loss" in Susan L. Greenblatt (ed.) *Providing Services for People with Sight Loss: A Multidisciplinary Perspective* Lexington, MA: Resources for Rehabilitation

Resources for I and R Specialists

Alliance of Information and Referral Systems (AIRS)
Box 3546
Joliet, IL 60434
(815) 744-6922

AIRS is a membership organization of I and R specialists in both public and private organizations. Publishes a "Directory of I and R Services in the U.S. and Canada." Annual journal, "Information and Referral," and "AIRS Newsletter" (5 issues per year). Individual professional membership, $50.00; institutions, sliding scale based on annual I and R program budget.

United Way of America
701 North Fairfax Street
Alexandria, VA 22314-2045
(703) 836-7100

United Way/Centraide Canada
600-150 Kent
Ottawa, Ontario K1P 5P4 Canada
(613) 236-7041

VISION Foundation, Inc.
818 Mt. Auburn Street
Watertown, MA 02172
(617) 926-4232   In MA, (800) 852-3029

The Role of the Family in the Adjustment to Blindness or Visual Impairment

James W. Warnke, A.C.S.W.

The various conditions that cause blindness or visual impairment, whether congenital or adventitious, affect not only the individuals themselves, but also members of their families. While it is true that professional interventions are directed toward the individuals who have experienced vision loss, it must be clearly understood that the larger context of the adjustment process is always a family affair. It is my opinion that the single most important factor predicting whether an individual's adjustment to vision loss will be successful or not is the capacity of the individual's family to adjust. This chapter will discuss the special role of families in the adjustment to blindness or visual impairment, so that members of the various helping professions can enhance their own effectiveness in this process.

Stages of Adjustment in Families

When blindness or visual impairment affects one family member, other family members often respond initially with a combination of fear, disbelief, anxiety, depression, rage, and paralysis. The initial reaction period can last in duration from days to years. Family members struggle to understand and adapt to the traumatic event that has occurred. They seek to understand what has happened and who or what is responsible; the implications of blindness or visual impairment for the individual; and the effects on the functioning of the family.

In many instances, family members have never met a person who is blind or visually impaired; the affected family member is the first

Susan L. Greenblatt, (ed.) *Meeting the Needs of People with Vision Loss: A Multidisciplinary Perspective,* Lexington, MA: Resources for Rehabilitation person that they know with a visual impairment. Lack of contact with other individuals who are blind or visually impaired may cause the family to feel a sense of isolation that can be overwhelming. Perceptions of the world and its effects on the family can change dramatically, with the sense of physical security and safety seriously eroded.

These initial reactions to vision loss may be understood through the questions that family members themselves ask:

• "If blindness or visual impairment can affect my father, mother, sister, brother, or child, what will happen to me?"

• "How can I feel safe and secure any longer in a world where my loved one loses his or her vision?"

• "What awful things may happen next?"

• "How will father or mother continue in his or her role as parent, breadwinner, nurturer, etc.?"

• "How will my child grow up to be a normal adult who is able to function independently?"

While these questions and a host of others may be at either the conscious or subconscious level, undoubtedly they occur whenever a family member is diagnosed as having serious vision loss (or any other seriously disabling condition) that cannot be corrected with surgery or other medical procedures. Children whose parents have become blind or visually impaired may become fearful of their own physical integrity. Parents of a child who is blind or visually impaired may become overly concerned and anxious about the well-being of this child as well as their other children.

The prognosis of irreversible vision loss often creates a sense of confusion in families, leading to a period of immobility. The exact etiology of the medical condition may be unclear, inconclusive, or poorly understood. Information about the types of assistance that are available may also be unclear or not provided at all (Greenblatt: 1988; 1989). It is a time when families frequently become immobilized, because they have no clearly defined goals and no information about how to get help. They may spend a great deal of psychic energy and valuable time worrying and grieving, with no inkling of how to improve the situation.

Fortunately, in most cases, a period of mobilization follows the period of immobilization. During this period, family members begin to take the first tentative actions required to assist the individual in his or her adjustment to blindness or visual impairment. The affected individual or another family member must reach the realization that vision loss has affected many other individuals and that there must be some means of support and training. This realization serves as the motivation to seek out services.

The effort to obtain services is not easy and produces its own psychological effects. Outreach to medical, educational, rehabilitation, and social service professionals requires assertiveness, perseverance, and a refusal to be intimidated by bureaucratic procedures. Since not all individuals have these characteristics, making these contacts may be quite difficult. Even individuals who are normally comfortable contacting professionals and government agencies on behalf of others may have difficulty when they are seeking information for themselves or for family members. Furthermore, contacting rehabilitation agencies indicates an acceptance that the vision loss is irreversible. Reaching the stage of acceptance requires going through a grieving process and perhaps denial. Therefore, these first steps are often tentative, hesitant, and fraught with anxiety and uncertainty.

The small successes gained in the mobilization period serve as encouragement to pursue services that lead to adjustment and movement back into the mainstream. Failures in the attempt to obtain information or services become temporary roadblocks. The successes and failures of the mobilization period are used as benchmarks by families in steering their course towards adaptation and adjustment. Progress in education, rehabilitation, orientation and mobility, and psychological adjustment allows the family to begin to think beyond the disability. In short, enough adjustment is achieved so that the larger issues of individual and family life may now be addressed.

The final phase is normalization, during which the family has thoroughly re-integrated the affected family member into the family structure and has re-integrated itself as a family into the community. The family that never reaches the normalization phase often becomes dysfunctional and relationships break down. Without professional intervention, divorce and substance abuse may occur.

Issues That Families Must Face

The first major issue that families confront when blindness or severe visual impairment occurs is the deep sense of loss and change. Parents joyfully expecting the birth of a healthy child, who are told by the pediatrician that their child has been born totally blind or with a severe visual impairment, must mourn the loss of the "ideal child" that they had hoped for. They must learn to accept and love the child who is blind or visually impaired. The adult offspring of a mother who becomes blind or visually impaired at age 77 must, in a very real psychological sense, mourn the loss of the sighted mother they have always known in order to accept, love, and support the mother who is now blind. Vision loss adds an extra dimension to the care of aging parents. Adult offspring of elders who are blind or visually impaired may be concerned that their parents will not be able to live in their own homes or care for themselves.

The psychological mourning process involves the full range of the cycle of denial, anger, depression, bargaining, and acceptance that has been suggested by Kubler-Ross (1969) in her work on death and dying. The more successfully families proceed through the mourning process, the better the prognosis for the eventual adjustment and adaptation for the individual who is blind or visually impaired and for the family's healthy functioning as a unit. The psychological mourning process is difficult when the affected family member and other family members proceed through the cycles at different speeds.

Families must learn how to share the practical, psychological, and financial requirements of assisting the affected individual in the adjustment process. Parents must educate themselves about the special developmental needs of their infant and find ways to meet these needs. Parents of school-age children may become preoccupied with developing and monitoring the special plans required to provide an appropriate education for their child. The anxieties, trials, and tribulations of adolescence can be significantly exacerbated and prolonged when issues of separation and individuation, sexual maturity, and burgeoning independence are complicated by the prolonged need for dependence upon parents.

Parents must not ignore the needs of other children in the family in their efforts to help the affected child. Siblings may experience embarrassment, jealousy, or rejection by their peers (Resources for Rehabilitation: 1991) when their sister or brother is blind or visually impaired. Siblings who plan to have children may seek genetic counseling to determine the inheritance patterns of the eye disease or condition.

Blindness or visual impairment may precipitate role reversals in the family. For example, when a spouse loses a job due to blindness or visual impairment, the other spouse may need to work to support the family. Adult offspring of aging parents who have experienced significant vision loss may be overwhelmed by the complex needs of parents who were previously perceived as competent, independent, and self-reliant. Vision loss may cause elders to feel frightened, disoriented, and helpless in the initial stages of adjustment. As sighted children of parents who are blind or visually impaired move into early and middle adulthood, they face special concerns about their roles as caretakers of their aging parents.

Family therapy, individual or group counseling, and support groups are resources to which family members may turn for help in resolving their feelings about blindness and visual impairment; their own anxieties, fears, and guilt; and ways to help the affected family member cope.

Patterns of Family Responses

There are many styles of adjustment that families manifest with regard to blindness and visual impairment. The healthiest forms of adjustment are generally characterized by responses in the family that are balanced. The frustrations of coping with and adjusting to blindness or visual impairment are not too deep, too prolonged, or too disorganizing either to the individual or to the family unit.

The *well-balanced family* is characterized by a capacity for empathy, support, flexibility, and the ability to acquire and utilize new information. Family members who are empathetic understand, appreciate, and communicate effectively their feelings and emotions. These are families where feelings are communicated clearly; where this communication is valued; and where the family responds to individual members' needs and feelings in a loving and compassionate way. The support that these families provide to a member who is blind or visually impaired is similar to the support that they provide to any family member in need. Well-balanced families also respond in a way that is flexible. Their modus operandi is to try a variety of methods to achieve a healthy adjustment; if adjustment cannot be achieved by one means, another means can and will be found.

Families that respond in a well-balanced way also demonstrate a capacity to acquire and to utilize new knowledge. In the case of blindness or visual impairment, this is knowledge about how people with vision loss function; the particular needs of the affected individual in the adjustment process; and how various members of the family can help. These families are skillful at networking with appropriate community and self-help resources. Ultimately, the family that responds in a well-balanced way to the trauma of blindness or visual impairment moves from the initial phase of shock and paralysis, to mobilization, and finally to a high degree of normalization and functioning in the mainstream.

Less helpful styles of response occur when families become stuck or fixated in one of the phases of the adjustment process or when a very unbalanced response pattern develops. One such pathological style may be characterized as the *paralyzed* family. This family has not adequately recovered from the initial shock of vision loss. The frustration that ensues is too deep and too disorganizing to overcome quickly or thoroughly. Paralyzed families are frequently but not exclusively families in which other serious traumas or disorganizing events have occurred, besides blindness or visual impairment. In this type of family, members seem overwhelmed, preoccupied, and unable to effectively help either themselves or each other in mastering the tasks of adjustment and adaptation. These families often exhibit difficulty in accepting or utilizing assistance offered by professionals and sometimes, without intending it, exhibit a chronic sense of frustration and helplessness.

The *over-protective family* mobilizes to protect and defend the member who is blind or visually impaired. This response often extends to protecting and defending the individual against the necessary and normal struggles in the process of adjustment, education, and rehabilitation. These families are characterized by a preoccupation with doing things *for* the member who is blind or visually impaired, rather than enabling the individual to do things for himself or herself. Frequently these families are resistant or overtly hostile and aggressive towards professionals who seek to enable the individual to become more self-sufficient. Enabling the individual family member who is blind or visually impaired to become independent would disrupt the family's need to perform the activities *for* the individual. In this case, the disability reinforces the family's pathological structure.

Ambivalence is another type of response exhibited by some families. This type of response occurs frequently, although not exclusively, in families of individuals who have a good deal of functional vision. In these families, there is a vacillation between over- and under-protection, over- and under-support, over- and under-estimation of capabilities and the impact of the vision loss on day-to-day functioning. These families are frequently highly functional in a practical sense, while on an emotional and psychological level, they experience tension and distress. Ambivalence may be exacerbated when vision loss is progressive or when visual functioning fluctuates. Individuals with vision loss caused by diabetes, for example, may find that their vision fluctuates during the course of one day. Individuals with progressive eye diseases or fluctuating vision find that not only is their vision "in limbo," (Oehler-Giarratana and Fitzgerald: 1980) but their emotions are as well. Families are also in limbo emotionally, and frequent trips to doctors' offices cause increased anxiety.

In paralyzed, over-protective, and ambivalent families, basic structural problems that existed prior to the onset of blindness or visual impairment must be worked out if the affected individual is expected to function independently. Failure to deal with problems in the family's basic structure may result in the disability feeding into the pathological needs of the family and prevent the individual from achieving a successful adaptation.

43

The Role of Professionals

When a family member must adjust to blindness or visual impairment, the appropriate role of the family unit is to provide physical and emotional environments that are empathetic, supportive, flexible, and open to new and important information. Professionals must focus not only on the individual who has experienced vision loss but also on the family as a whole. The goal is to help the family become the most empathetic, supportive, flexible, and understanding unit that it is capable of becoming. The family can then become the vehicle in which the individual moves from the original traumatic experience of vision loss to normalization.

In addition to providing competent and compassionate services in their specialty areas, all professionals must provide a point of entry into the larger system of services. For example, it is essential that ophthalmologists know about the rehabilitation and special education services that are available in their geographical area and to develop personal relationships with the in-take staff of those agencies.

When an ophthalmologist refers a patient for services, he or she can then describe the services offered by the agency, thereby ameliorating the patient's anxieties and maximizing the probability that the patient will follow up on the referral. Simply informing the patient that such a service exists or handing the patient or accompanying family member a phone number is not usually sufficient incentive, especially at the time of the initial diagnosis. At follow-up appointments, the ophthalmologist should ask if contacts have been made with referral agencies or professionals and if so, what the outcome was.

In the same way, special educators and rehabilitation professionals need to have a basic familiarity with the routine manifestations of anxiety, depression, and symptoms of significant family dysfunction in order to make appropriate referrals for mental health services. Psychotherapists must have a knowledge of conditions that cause blindness or visual impairment in order for psychotherapy with families in transition to be successful. Psychotherapists working with this population must have ongoing consultations with ophthalmologists in order to understand the physiology of the eye condition, the effects of treatment, and the physical and functional effects of the disease.

Conclusion

When families are able to go through the normal grieving process along with the family member who has experienced blindness or visual impairment, both the family and the individual will benefit. In healthy families, the ability to cope successfully with a devastating experience serves to strengthen the family unit and prepare its members for future crises. Obtaining information about the opportunities for rehabilitation and ultimate independence for individuals who are blind or visually impaired contributes to a restored sense of physical and psychological security.

References

Greenblatt, Susan L.
1989   "The Need for Coordinated Care" pp. 25-37 in Susan L. Greenblatt (ed.) *Providing Services for People with Vision Loss: A Multidisciplinary Perspective* Lexington, MA: Resources for Rehabilitation
1988   "Physicians and Chronic Impairment: A Study of Ophthalmologists' Interactions with Visually Impaired and Blind Patients" *Social Science and Medicine* 26:393-399

Kubler-Ross, Elisabeth
1969   *On Death and Dying* New York, NY: Macmillan Company

Oehler-Giarratana, Judith and Roy G. Fitzgerald
1980   "Group Therapy with Blind Diabetics" *Archives of General Psychiatry* 37 (Apr):4:463-467

Resources for Rehabilitation
1991   *Resources for People with Disabilities and Chronic Conditions* Lexington, MA: Resources for Rehabilitation

Special Populations

Diabetes and Vision Loss: Special Considerations

Marla Bernbaum, M.D.

Diabetes mellitus is the leading cause of blindness in the United States for individuals between the ages of 20 and 74 years. Approximately 5,800 cases of new blindness each year are attributable to the disease (Harris and Hamman: 1985). The population of persons diagnosed with diabetes in the United States is estimated at 6.8 million (U.S. Department of Health and Human Services: 1990). This figure is doubled when undiagnosed cases are also considered. Twelve percent of insulin-dependent individuals who have had diabetes for more than thirty years are blind. Approximately 22% of all patients with diabetes have some degree of vision impairment and 5% have severe impairment. Diabetic retinopathy is the major cause of vision loss; however, glaucoma and cataracts occur with increased frequency and at earlier ages in persons with diabetes than in the rest of the population. Ninety-seven percent of insulin-treated individuals and 80% of individuals with diabetes who do not require insulin have retinopathy after 15 years. Approximately 40% of insulin-treated and 5% of non-insulin-treated individuals with diabetes develop advanced proliferative retinopathy (Kline: 1985).

The nonproliferative form of the disease or "background retinopathy" usually does not result in significant vision impairment but is detectible during an ophthalmological examination. There is an alteration of the small vessels nourishing the retina, resulting in small out-pouchings (micro-aneurisms), with leakage of fluid and blood. Hemorrhages and deposits, called exudates, may be visible on the retina. In some cases, fluid accumulation around the macula can result in moderate vision impairment, with acuities ranging from 20/40 to 20/200. This condition, known as macular edema, is very difficult to treat but does not progress to total blindness (Fleischmann: 1987). Klein et al. (1989) recently

Susan L. Greenblatt, (ed.) Meeting the Needs of People with Vision Loss: A Multidisciplinary Perspective, Lexington, MA: Resources for Rehabilitation

reported an 8.2 to 8.4% incidence of macular edema among participants taking insulin in the Wisconsin Epidemiological Study of Diabetic Retinopathy. The incidence was 2.9% for participants not taking insulin. Macular edema may improve with laser photocoagulation therapy if treated early in its course.

Proliferative retinopathy is a more advanced form of the disease, in which new fragile blood vessels are formed. These vessels grow out of the surface of the retina into the vitreous body and are easily ruptured. The resulting hemorrhages can cause sudden occlusion of vision. Eventually, there is shrinking and fibrosis of vessels and membranous materials, resulting in traction detachments and scarring of the retina. This form of retinopathy may be marked by a fluctuating course, with sudden devastating hemorrhage, slow resolution of blood, and permanent retinal damage. Early treatment of proliferative retinopathy with panretinal photocoagulation therapy results in a 50% decrease in vision loss. Vitrectomy, in which hemorrhage-containing vitreous is removed from the eye, and surgical repair of the retina may help to restore visual function (Fleischmann: 1987; Klein: 1985).

Vision loss in diabetes correlates with the duration of the disease. It has been suggested that tight control of the blood sugar and possibly the blood pressure may prevent development and progression of diabetic retinopathy (Klein: 1985, 1989). Although it is recommended that patients with diabetes strive for the best possible control, prevention of diabetic eye disease has not yet been possible. Sophisticated treatment for other complications of diabetes, such as serious infection and heart and renal failure, has increased the probability of prolonged survival for persons with diabetes. As a result, there is an increase in the number of individuals requiring rehabilitation services for severe vision impairment or blindness. Appropriate rehabilitation programs require an integrated multidisciplinary approach to address medical care, special psychosocial considerations, and accommodation of physical limitations imposed by concurrent diabetic complications.

Special Psychosocial Considerations

All persons with new and chronic vision loss must learn to cope with the emotional and physical stresses of the condition. When severe vision impairment is superimposed upon diabetes mellitus, there are additional psychosocial ramifications that must be addressed. Diabetes is a progressive systemic disease, characterized by potential life-threatening complications and early mortality. Patients are asked to play a major role in the management of their illness through administration of daily insulin and other medications, self-monitoring of blood sugars, and adherence to specific dietary and exercise regimens. The inability of the individual to participate in the self-care plan may lead to acute symptoms of illness associated with poor diabetic control and to advancement of chronic complications.

Conventional diabetes self-management requires adequate visual acuity and coordination. Insulin must be drawn into a finely marked syringe. Blood sugar monitoring requires placement of a small droplet of blood on a tiny reagent strip. Results are obtained either by comparing the reacted reagent strip to a color chart or by placement of the strip in a meter that generates a digital display. Dietary compliance may depend on the ability to read food labels and to weigh and measure food portions. Patients with failing vision who have not been trained in adaptive skills will inevitably become dependent on friends and family members for this basic personal care. Since insulin administration, blood sugar monitoring, and meal-times must be carefully coordinated, the loss of independence is further hindered because the individual must alter lifestyle and routines to match the schedule of the care-giver. The result is frustration, depression, loss of self-esteem and additional stress on the interpersonal relationships with family and friends. Early intervention and training with adaptive equipment for diabetes self-management may alleviate a great deal of daily stress by restoring independence and self-care (Bernbaum et al.: 1988a, 1989a).

Heart disease, peripheral vascular disease, kidney disease, and nerve disease may occur concurrently with the loss of vision. In some cases, these complications may have progressed to seriously disabling, even life-threatening stages prior to the onset of vision impairment. In other cases, vision loss may be the heralding event triggering the patient's awareness of vulnerability to other potentially devastating complications. The presence of multiple complications may be physically and psychologically overwhelming, and even the realization of the numerous potential complications may be paralyzing. The sense of hopelessness and depression may totally impede the ability of the individual to respond to any rehabilitative assistance that is offered.

Diabetic retinopathy often results in long periods of fluctuating vision. Participants in one study demonstrated low levels of self-esteem and psychosocial well-being through self-rating questionnaires. Subjects with fluctuating vision had significantly higher levels of depression when compared to subjects with stable vision, even though the latter had poorer visual acuity (Bernbaum et al.: 1988b). Fluctuating vision can also lead to increased levels of frustration and anxiety with alternating periods of optimism and pessimism regarding the final visual outcome. As a result, these individuals may be reluctant to pursue a rehabilitation program until it is certain that normal functional vision will not be regained. In these instances, counseling should stress the physical and emotional benefits of rehabilitation training, while helping the individual work through the fears and anxiety associated with the uncertainty of improvement (Oehler-Giarratana: 1978).

Diabetes, failing vision, and other disabling complications in one family member are likely to have a serious impact on family dynamics. There may be enormous social and financial burdens that the family is not equipped to handle. The psychotherapists and a social worker, who may act as case manager, will need to address these issues with the individual and the family through coordinated counseling and support services.

The complexity of the psychological and social issues that confront the individual and the family when severe vision loss occurs in the setting of diabetes mellitus requires in-depth understanding of both conditions. Referrals should be made to psychotherapists and social workers who have adequate knowledge and expertise to address the compounded problems. Peer support groups can be useful to dissipate social isolation and create an empathetic atmosphere for ventilation and problem solving (Oehler-Giarratana: 1980; Tattersan et al.: 1985).

Special Aspects of Rehabilitation

Rehabilitation programs designed to promote independence for patients with diabetes and vision loss will need to focus on several aspects unique to the diabetic patient: (1) training in diabetes self-care skills and (2) consideration of physical limitations associated with acute and chronic complications of diabetes mellitus.

An early component of the rehabilitation program should include an introduction to adaptive devices for insulin administration and blood sugar monitoring. A variety of syringe magnifiers are available for individuals with adequate functional vision. For those with no functional vision, pre-cut gauges and adjustable devices that fit standard syringes can be obtained for accurate dose measurement. Clicking tactile pens with pre-filled insulin cartridges are now readily available through most pharmacies and suppliers of diabetic equipment. Several blood sugar monitoring systems, adapted with speech synthesizers, allow independent blood sugar measurement. Individuals should be referred to a qualified diabetes educator who can assess individual needs and abilities and aid in the selection of appropriate devices. A diabetes educator familiar with the nuances of self-management skills for individuals with vision loss can ensure proper training for confidence and accuracy in technique. Individuals with diabetes should receive routine ADL (Activities of Daily Living) training in food preparation, with emphasis on avoidance of practices that may result in cuts and burns. Minimal injuries to the skin, if unattended, may result in serious infections in individuals with diabetes.

Physicians will usually refer patients with diabetes to a dietician who may instruct them to select meals from a diabetes exchange list or from a renal diet plan. There may be additional restrictions, such as limitations on cholesterol or salt. For patients with poor vision, instructions should be recorded on a cassette which can be substituted for the usual written materials. Recorded and braille versions of the standard diabetes exchange diet are available. Individuals may require specific training in tactile methods for estimating portion size and for the use of tactile scales and measuring utensils (Bernbaum et al.: 1988a, 1989a).

There are numerous precautions that orientation and mobility instructors should take with individuals who have diabetes. Exercise can induce low blood sugar reactions in persons treated with insulin or oral blood sugar-lowering medications. Individuals who have been inactive prior to beginning mobility training may experience unexpected drops in the blood sugar, even with low to moderate levels of activity. Since medication action is planned to match food ingestion, mobility lessons should be scheduled to avoid delay or omission of routine meals. The client or the instructor should carry a source of readily available carbohydrate. Suitable items include small cans or cartons of juice, hard candy, or glucose tablets. If the client exhibits signs of low blood sugar, i.e., weakness, tremors, profuse sweating, loss of coordination, confusion, or inappropriate emotion, he or she should be encouraged to eat one of these foods. The lesson should not be resumed until the symptoms have completely resolved. When experiencing excessively high blood sugar, some individuals with diabetes may feel fatigued or have difficulty concentrating. Other patients will have no obvious symptoms and will have no problems in proceeding with the planned session.

Individuals may be limited in their ability to participate in mobility training due to heart, kidney, peripheral vascular, or nerve disease that frequently co-exist with failing vision. These complications, individually or in combination, can predispose individuals to fatigue and generalized weakness. Nerve disease, known as diabetic neuropathy, may lead to poor sensation in the hands and feet and poor balance. Training in potentially dangerous settings, such as stairways without adequate railings, is inadvisable. Neuropathy involving the feet, combined with circulatory problems, places individuals at high risk for injury to the feet that may in turn result in serious infections or amputations. When long mobility sessions are planned, it is essential that people with neuropathy of the feet wear protective, comfortable, and properly-fitted footwear. Scrapes and cuts that do occur should be closely monitored for signs of infection.

Loss of sensation and muscle weakness in the hands may limit tactile ability and fine motor skills. This occurs most often in older individuals but can occur in younger persons. Consequently, tactile skills managed easily by other blind individuals may be acquired more slowly and awkwardly by individuals with diabetes. Braille reading, for example, may be difficult or impossible for some individuals (Heinrichs and Moorhouse: 1968). However, even individuals with objective evidence of advanced nerve disease have learned to master jumbo braille when sufficiently motivated (Bernbaum et al.: 1989b). No one with diabetes should be discouraged from at least attempting to learn braille, a skill which can provide an added measure of independence and recreational pleasure. Fortunately, many resource and recreational materials are also readily available in large print and audiocassette formats.

Unfortunately, interruptions in the rehabilitation program frequently occur. As diabetic retinopathy advances, intermittent surgical intervention may be required. Concurrent illness and convalescence associated with other complications may impede progress. The rehabilitation plan may need to be modified to accommodate alterations in physical ability. The rehabilitation team should maintain contact with the physician and other medical care providers so that anticipated interruptions and changes in status can be dealt with effectively. Input from the health care team and psychotherapists is essential in designing an appropriate rehabilitation plan.

Multidisciplinary Approach

A special rehabilitation program for individuals with diabetes and vision impairment was piloted at St. Louis University (Bernbaum et al.: 1988a, 1989a). Physicians and nurse specialists, exercise specialists, and psychologists worked closely with rehabilitation professionals to design a comprehensive program. Prior to the initiation of the program, all staff members attended a workshop presented by a rehabilitation teacher and an orientation and mobility instructor. The workshop included sighted guide technique and sensitivity training. Participants, referred by physicians, nurses and local rehabilitation agencies, came to the program center three half-days per week for twelve weeks. Many of the participants were simultaneously enrolled in standard rehabilitation programs. Schedules were coordinated by rehabilitation service case managers.

Each half-day session included an exercise period followed by an educational session (twice weekly) or a support group meeting (once weekly). The exercise routine consisted of ten-minute group warm-up and cool-down periods and a 20 to 40 minute aerobic phase, during which participants exercised at their own pace, through stationary bicycling, walking, and rowing. (Aerobic exercise is sustained repetitive activity which builds strength and endurance for the muscles and heart.) Blood sugar levels, pulse rates, and blood pressures were measured at regular intervals throughout the exercise session. All participants underwent a medical evaluation with assessments of heart function and exercise endurance prior to entering the program. Exercise routines were modified according to these factors, and the length and intensity of the activity was gradually increased, as tolerated, over the twelve weeks. A guide-rope was strung along an indoor track to allow blind participants to walk independently. Warm-up and cool-down stretching and toning exercises were largely performed sitting in a straight-back chair to avoid forward bending of the head below the level of the heart. Bending forward, excessive bouncing, and heavy weight lifting were avoided, since these activities may aggravate retinopathy.

Educational sessions were conducted in an informal, interactive group setting. The curriculum sequentially addressed: (1) general aspects of diabetes such as symptoms of high and low blood sugar, treatment, complications, and preventative care; (2) discussion and demonstration of techniques and devices for diabetes self-care for individuals who are visually impaired; (3) precautions for exercising safely with a focus on special needs due to diabetes, visual impairment, and other complications, as well as instruction in appropriate monitoring of blood sugar and pulse rate during exercise at home; and (4) nutritional education concerning general principles of the diabetic diet and menu planning, as well as demonstration of adaptive kitchen utensils used for measuring food portions and ensuring safety during food preparation. Discussions were led respectively by a physician, a diabetes educator, an exercise specialist, and a dietician. The diabetes educator and dietician also met with each participant as often as necessary, providing individualized hands-on instruction and menu planning. All essential information was pre-recorded on audiocassettes for home reference, and individualized dietary instructions were recorded for each person.

Support group topics addressed difficulties in coping with diabetes and blindness, effects on interpersonal relations and social interactions, personal losses, and emotional responses such as fear, frustration, depression, and guilt. Participants were encouraged to share negative and positive experiences and their own resolutions to specific problems. A staff psychologist was available to provide individual counseling as needed.

The professional staff and the participants enthusiastically embraced the program, and many of the participants continue to return to ongoing support groups. Objective data obtained over a three-year period revealed significant improvements for participants in parameters reflecting diabetes control, physical endurance, and psychological adaptation. All of the participants in this program were between the ages of 21 and 72 years, spanning the years in which diabetic retinopathy is most prevalent. The ability of older patients to respond to such a program is uncertain and requires assessment of individual physical and cognitive status. A few of the older persons in this pilot program were able to benefit from exercise and group support but were unable to master some aspects of diabetes self-management independently, despite intensive instruction.

Since diabetic retinopathy rarely begins to develop until after puberty, there is little experience involving children and adolescents, Children with other causes of blindness may develop diabetes coincidently and would require a rehabilitation plan including instruction in self-management skills. This is essential for independent function. Appropriate timing for this instruction will depend on the dexterity and emotional maturity of the child. Thus, persons of certain age groups as well as those with severe physical disabilities may not be able to participate in all aspects of this comprehensive program. However, selected elements of the program may be applicable and easily reproduced at other centers.

Conclusion

Clearly, the individual with diabetes and vision impairment has a unique blend of medical, psychosocial, and rehabilitation needs. A proper balance of therapy, support, and rehabilitation must be provided by an integrated team of professionals. It may be critical to enlist the services of a social worker who can act as the case manager to ensure that the individual gains access to necessary medical care, psychological counseling, and rehabilitation services. Most individuals with diabetes are under the care of a physician when the vision impairment is first detected. Referral to an ophthalmologist is routine. The services of a diabetes educator and dietician are usually coordinated through the physician's office or clinic. A certified diabetes educator is a nurse or other allied health professional who has training and experience in teaching self-care skills to persons with diabetes. Diabetes educators often work in conjunction with physicians who specialize in treating diabetes, or they are available to teach patients in hospitals or out-patient clinic settings. (A few rehabilitation agencies employ diabetes educators specifically to instruct clients in adaptive self-care skills.)

Unfortunately, many health care providers are unaware of rehabilitation services available to their patients. (See Weisse: 1989 for a description of rehabilitation services.) Also psychotherapists and social workers who might bridge the gap between medical and rehabilitation services may not be sought until the vision impairment is overtly disabling and the psychosocial dysfunction is unmanageable to the patient and the family. Once appropriate referrals are made, rehabilitation professionals often lack access to the medical professionals and may have an inadequate understanding of their client's physical abilities and limitations.

There is a great need for multidisciplinary workshops and programs such as the St. Louis University rehabilitation program. Medical professionals need education regarding general rehabilitation services and adaptive devices for diabetes self-management. They need training in sighted guide technique and other skills that will allow them to interact more effectively with visually impaired patients. Rehabilitation counselors and teachers need to understand the complexities of their clients' illness and also need updated information on adaptive equipment for persons with diabetes and vision loss. Task forces have recently been created by several diabetes and blindness advocacy groups to address the need for greater integration of the disciplines.* There has been some sharing of resources and a few guidelines have been issued. An increasing interest in the problem has been expressed in the professional and consumer literature. Hopefully, in ensuing years more efforts will be focused on accommodating the growing needs of individuals with diabetes and visual impairment.

* Committee for the Visually Impaired, American Association of Diabetes Educators, Cleveland Sight Center, 1909 East 101 Street, Cleveland, OH 44106

References

Bernbaum, Marla, Stewart G. Albert, Stephanie R. Brusca, Ami Drimmer, and Paul N. Duckro
1988a "Promoting Diabetes Self-Management and Independence in the Visually Impaired: A Model Clinical Program" *The Diabetes Educator* 14: 51-54

Bernbaum, Marla, Stewart G. Albert, and Paul N. Duckro
1988b "Profiles in Patients With Visual Impairment Due to Diabetic Retinopathy" *Diabetes Care* 11: 551-557

Bernbaum, Marla, Stewart G. Albert, Stephanie R. Brusca, Ami Drimmer, Paul N. Duckro, Jerome D. Cohen, Mario C. Trindade, and Alan B. Silverburg
1989a "A Model Clinical Program for Patients With Diabetes and Vision Impairment" *The Diabetes Educator* 15: 325-330

Bernbaum, Marla, Stewart G. Albert, and John D. McGarry
1989b "Diabetic Neuropathy and Braille Ability" *Archives of Neurology* 47: 1179-1181

Fleischmann, Jay A.
1987 "How Retinopathy Develops" *Juvenile Diabetes Foundation International Countdown* 8:20

Harris, Maureen I., and Richard F. Hamman, (eds.)
1985 *Diabetes in America* U.S. Department of Health and Human Services, NIH Publication No. 85-1468: 1-6

Heinrichs, R.W., and J.A. Moorhouse
1968   "Touch Perception Thresholds in Blind Diabetic Subjects in Relation to the Reading of Braille Type" *Diabetes* 17: 302

Klein, Ronald, and Barbara E. K. Klein
1985   "Vision Disorders in Diabetes" pp 1-6 in Maureen I. Harris and Richard F. Hamman (eds.) *Diabetes in America* U.S. Department of Health and Human Services, NIH Publication No. 85-1468

Klein, Ronald, Scot E. Moss, Barbara E. K. Klein, Matthew D. Davis, and David L. DeMets
1989   "The Wisconsin Epidemiologic Study of Diabetic Retinopathy" *Ophthalmology* 96: 1501-1510

Oehler-Giarratana, Judith
1978   "Meeting the Psychosocial and Rehabilitative Needs of the Visually Impaired Diabetic" *Journal of Visual Impairment and Blindness* 72: 358-361

Oehler-Giarratana, Judith and Roy G. Fitzgerald
1980   "Group Therapy With Blind Diabetics" *Archives of General Psychiatry* 37:(Apr)4:463-467

Tattersall, Robert B., David K. McCulloch, and Mark Aveline
1985   "Group Therapy in the Treatment of Diabetes" *Diabetes Care* 8: 180-188

U.S. Department of Health and Human Services
1990   *Diabetes Surveillance 1980-1987* Public Health Service, Centers for Disease Control, Center for Chronic Disease Prevention and Health Promotion, April, Atlanta

Weisse, Fran A.
1989   "Making Referrals for Rehabilitation" pp. 56-71 in Susan L. Greenblatt (ed.) *Providing Services for People with Vision Loss: A Multidisciplinary Perspective* Lexington, MA: Resources for Rehabilitation

Special Needs of Children and Adolescents

James W. Warnke, A.C.S.W.

Working with children and adolescents who are blind or visually impaired requires great skill and sensitivity. Perhaps the most important concept in working with youngsters who are blind or visually impaired is to think in terms of developmental stages. Understanding the developmental norms appropriate to children of different ages is a prerequisite in helping youngsters overcome or compensate for the invariable developmental lags precipitated by blindness or visual impairment. A familiarity with literature such as Erikson's (1975; 1977; 1985) work on psychological development in the stages of childhood development; Piaget's (1948; 1953) seminal works on cognitive development in childhood; Kohlberg's (1984) study of moral development in children; and Thomas and Chess' (1977) study of temperamental styles in children form the backdrop necessary to understand the needs of children who are blind or visually impaired. The knowledge of developmental stages is crucial in determining the appropriate language to use, the level of concepts the child understands, and realistic expectations of responsibility.

Stress

Youngsters who are blind or visually impaired are under chronic stress, caused by the need to overcome or compensate for the deprivations caused by blindness or visual impairment. Children who are blind or visually impaired must process with four senses what sighted children process with five. Children who must function with one less sense intact are subject to more stress and strain than children who have all five senses functioning normally. Therefore, these children are in need of more routine counseling and assistance than children with all five senses intact.

Susan L. Greenblatt, (ed.) Meeting the Needs of People with Vision Loss: A Multidisciplinary Perspective, Lexington, MA: Resources for Rehabilitation

The extra energy required for orientation and mobility skills, increased demands on memory, and the simple need for more time to accomplish routine tasks are not beyond the capacities of most children and adolescents who are blind or visually impaired, but they are routinely exhausting. The classic symptoms of stress and stress syndrome, including anxiety, periods of depression, a need for solitude, and occasional disturbances of sleep and appetite, are frequently noted in these youngsters and need to be understood and addressed by parents and professionals alike.

Special Educational Needs

The special educational needs of children who are blind or visually impaired are myriad. There is a growing body of literature in this area of special education, and departments of vocational rehabilitation are expressing an increased interest in this population group. Educational opportunities range from mainstream placements in regular classrooms with supportive services and adaptive devices, to more extensive support systems in resource room programs or self-contained classrooms, to more traditional residential schools for students who are blind. The idea that children and adolescents who are blind or visually impaired belong in the mainstream of education is a good one. It is crucial, however, that a high degree of cooperation and collaboration among professionals be established and maintained. The vision teacher, regular classroom teacher, and ophthalmologist must work together to assure that the student's needs are met. Where this collaboration does not occur, mainstreaming degenerates into a less expensive educational option and a rationalization for closing special placements for students who are blind or visually impaired.

An integral part of providing educational services is the development of an Individualized Education Plan (IEP), required by federal law in the United States. Legal rights include the right to appeal decisions and the right to bring professionals chosen by the parents to hearings. An IEP is a curriculum plan with adaptations pertinent to the child's specific needs, developed by special educators who work in the field of vision, school psychologists, regular classroom teachers, school administrators, and social workers in collaboration with parents.

Joint planning among a variety of professionals helps the child achieve realistic goals and also helps professionals fulfill their obligations. A case example illustrates this point. I recently attended an IEP meeting for a ten year old boy who had been a former psychotherapy client of mine. I was invited to the meeting to provide information about the developmental needs of children who are blind or visually impaired and to offer insights about my former client. Others attending the meeting included the principal of the elementary school, the present classroom teacher, the classroom teacher for the next school year, the psychologist who also served as the case manager for the school district, the physical education teacher, the art teacher, and the itinerant vision teacher. We discussed discipline, homework, how to adapt the art program, how to utilize the special physical education program more creatively, and plans for interactive socialization to help this youngster become an integral part of the new classroom setting. (A second meeting was to include the youngster's parents.) The meeting, which had begun with a sense of anticipation, anxiety, and frustration, contributed to the development of educational goals for this student and a plan to achieve those goals. Those attending the meeting felt calmer and more focused than they had prior to the meeting.

Socialization and Social Interaction

Just as there is a need within the educational setting for an Individualized Educational Plan, there is a need for an Individualized Empowerment Plan within the family. The family needs to pay particular attention to helping the youngster create and find opportunities for adequate and appropriate socialization and social experience.

Youngsters who are blind or visually impaired frequently need the assistance of adults so that they can interact with their peers and acquire the developmental benefits derived from participation in these activities. Although adult assistance may be necessary, parents must be careful not to be overly protective. By doing too much for their child, they will raise a child who is unable to act on his or her own and who fears independence.

Much social interaction among adults revolves around conversation, where ideas, thoughts, and experiences are shared. With children and adolescents, social interactions very often revolve around a special activity. In general, the younger the child, the more activity-oriented are the social interactions. Young children do not routinely talk together, they routinely play together. Theirs is a world of games and activities, fantasies, and projects.

Children learn who they are; they learn a sense of competence and well-being; and they learn to feel good about themselves by engaging in social activities. Children learn a variety of skills through the use of board games, word games, and video games; participation in these activities contributes to the development of self-esteem.

Virtually all of these activities require modification in order for youngsters who are blind or visually impaired to participate. These modifications may be technical, such as soccer balls that beep; magnifying or speech devices for computer screens that make video games accessible; or braille versions of Monopoly, Uno, and other games. Or the modifications may take the form of mediation by adults or older youth, who verbally describe the nonverbal portions of the activity and coach and encourage the youngster.

Adaptations for a 16 year old girl who is totally blind illustrate how adults can readily modify the social interactions of youngsters who are blind or visually impaired. Alice lived in a rural community and had few friends or social contacts until a school social worker referred her to an adult mentor for the youth organization at the girl's church. The mentor arranged a carpool with another family so that Alice would have transportation to meetings. He asked a member of the church who was an orientation and mobility instructor to speak to the group about blindness and visual impairment and to teach sighted guide techniques. Alice used her cassette tape recorder to keep a list of the members' telephone numbers and volunteered to call them to remind them about meetings. Alice's pleasant personality and willingness to work earned her rapid promotions in this organization. The result was an enhanced social network organized around tasks and activities as well as peers. A developing sense of social grace and competence for this young woman was the result of participation in these activities.

A 13 year old boy who is visually impaired and who also has serious hearing impairment was bullied at school. Jeff's inability to interpret verbal and nonverbal communication in its more subtle forms and his inability to participate in the athletics program were at the heart of his problems. In the small town where he lived, athletics were extremely important to both students and parents. Jeff voiced an interest in studying karate; his parents initially rejected this idea as unrealistic. A social worker involved with the case, located a karate school where the chief instructor, who was also a special education teacher, was able to address Jeff's special needs. Conferences with his parents, ophthalmologist, and audiologist delineated the particular karate activities that they thought should be permitted and those that should be avoided for his safety.

Participation in karate with his peers enhanced Jeff's sense of athletic competence. His self-esteem improved in a way that neither his parents nor his teachers had previously imagined possible. This experience also enabled his parents to permit Jeff to take part in a variety of other activities and to relinquish the role of overly protective parents.

Jeff's own request to study karate illustrates another important point. Youngsters who are blind or visually impaired should help to make decisions about their own life course, including decisions that may seem minor (such as participating in sports) to major decisions about educational plans and career options. Asking youngsters what they want to do or what they think they cannot do because of blindness or visual impairment enables parents and professionals to jointly devise strategies with the youngsters.

Adults who are blind or visually impaired are often willing to serve as role models or mentors for children and adolescents with vision loss. These adults show how they live and work independently; demonstrate their own use of adaptive aids; share practical information; provide emotional support; and encourage youngsters to participate in recreational and other activities.

Using Adaptive Aids

Parents and educators frequently complain that children and particularly teenagers resist the use of adaptive devices both in educational and social settings. Adolescents who are visually impaired are often able to improve their mobility and safety by using a white cane but refuse to do so. Children who receive recorded material and Talking Book machines often let them collect dust on a shelf or in the closet. Monoculars remain hidden in coat pockets, rather than used on the street. The use of closed circuit televisions frequently becomes the subject of discipline in the home, with parents insisting that they be used for homework.

Why do children and adolescents respond this way? Like adults, children and adolescents who are blind or visually impaired do not want to have a disability. Mastering the use of adaptive aids constitutes an admission of blindness or visual impairment to both oneself and to others. Adults who have diabetes often behave in a similar manner, by refusing to adhere to their special diets and insulin injection schedules. Rejection of the visible signs of illness or disability is a common and natural human behavior. During the teenage years in particular, the value placed on appearance is often paramount. It is more important to teenagers' self-esteem to appear normal than to use devices that improve functioning in school and other activities but make them appear different from their peers. Students are usually much more interested in the social dimensions of school than in studying. This is an important concept to keep in mind when working with children and particularly with adolescents.

A helpful technique in working with adolescents is to acknowledge that they will refuse to use adaptive devices now, but as they mature, the ability to function well will become more important than appearance, and these same youngsters will voluntarily use the devices. I recently told a 16 year old boy who is visually impaired that he could look forward to the time when it would be more important for him to see the chemistry notes on the blackboard than worrying that his peers would reject him because he used a monocular. While he received this suggestion with some skepticism, my experience over many years has taught me that he will change his mind.

It should be remembered, however, that children are indeed children, and that parents and teachers must at times require that children use their adaptive devices. Once children become accustomed to using their devices, their resistance will dissipate. Furthermore, if low vision aids and other adaptive devices are introduced early in the child's life, the devices become part of the child's identity. For example, when adaptive devices are introduced for recreational activities, children may view them favorably and show them off to their friends. A monocular may be used to spot the pins in a bowling alley; a speech synthesizer may be used to play a video game; or a closed circuit television system may be used to examine stamps or coins. Adaptive aids may be broken or lost more frequently by young children, but the benefits of using the aids outweigh the inconvenience and cost of replacements. It is important to remember that the way in which the aids are introduced to the child and the age at which they are introduced will have a profound impact on the child's acceptance or rejection of the aids.

Peer Interaction

It is important that youngsters who are blind or visually impaired develop a network of relationships with peers who have normal vision in order to participate in school and social activities and to prepare for life after schooling ends. It is equally important, particularly in this era of mainstreaming, that youngsters who are blind or visually impaired have an opportunity for social interaction with other youngsters who are blind or visually impaired. It is not uncommon for a youngster who is blind or visually impaired to be the only such student in a particular school district or in a particular school building. "Being the only one" of any category may be detrimental and foster a sense of isolation. Normal childhood and adolescent development requires that youngsters interact with other youngsters who are "just like them." I have frequently spoken with youngsters and adolescents who are mainstreamed in regular classrooms during the school year and attend special camp programs for youngsters who are blind or visually impaired during the summer. They routinely describe these summer camp experiences as some of the best times in their lives, where they can talk with others who have had similar experiences, anxieties, problems, and hopes, and where they learn that their difficulties are not unique. They discover that there are peers who can understand them in a way that no sighted peer can, because they have a bond of shared experiences.

Conclusion

Some families and professionals mistakenly carry the idea of normalization too far by evaluating successful adjustment to blindness or visual impairment on the basis of youngsters' abilities to function "as if they were sighted." Finding references to blindness and visual impairment upsetting or distasteful, families and professionals sometimes steer youngsters away from appropriate and useful interactions, organizations, and recreational, vocational, or educational experiences specifically geared to their disability group. It is my firm belief that this is a disservice to the youngsters involved.

Parents must accept their child's blindness or visual impairment and recognize that they must seek help to enable the child to reach his or her full potential just as they would if their child had other special needs. Although the guidelines parents use in raising a child who is blind or visually impaired are necessarily different than those used to raise a child with normal vision, they must avoid being overprotective.

Educators must work jointly with the child, parents, psychotherapists, rehabilitation specialists, and physicians to help determine a course of action that is healthy, safe, and contributes to the youngster's self-esteem and ability to function in society.

References

Erikson, Erik H.
1985   *Children and Society* New York, NY: Norton
1977   *Toys and Reasons: Stages in the Ritualization of Experience* New York, NY: Norton
1975   *Studies of Play* New York, NY: Arno Press

Kohlberg, Lawrence
1984   *The Psychology of Moral Development: The Nature and Validity of Moral Stages* San Francisco, CA: Harper and Row

Piaget, Jean
1953   *The Origin of Intelligence in the Child* London: Routledge and
        Paul
1948   *The Moral Judgement of the Child* Glencoe, IL: Free Press

Thomas, Alexander and Stella Chess
1977   *Temperament and Development* New York, NY: Brunner/Mazel

Older Adults with Vision and Hearing Losses*

Martha Bagley, M.S.

Susan is 78 years old and losing vision to age-related macular degeneration. She has needed a hearing aid for years but resisted getting one. After raising a large family she lived alone, caring for herself very well. Now her children tell her she is confused and can't cope. They want her to go to a nursing home. She doesn't want to because she doesn't feel sick. She believes there must be some way to keep doing the things she has always done.

Linda was admitted to a nursing home eight years ago after a severe fall. She is 75 and has diabetes and arthritis. When she arrived at the nursing home, her hearing was so poor that even when she could be persuaded to wear her hearing aid, it didn't help much. The staff communicated with her by writing notes in extra large letters; now she can barely read them. She is angry all of the time and shouts at everyone. If staff surprise her or touch her unexpectedly she is likely to hit them. Some of the staff want to send Linda to a special dementia unit; others refuse to even try to work with her. She spends a lot of time alone in her room in bed.

Mary is severely and profoundly retarded and has lived in a highly structured institutional setting for most of her 55 years. Staff have noticed a change in Mary's behavior recently. She seems more confused, at times refusing to respond and at other times overreacting. Mary has never had her hearing tested. When her vision was last tested, it was not corrected because, according to staff, "She can't read or drive anyway."

Susan L. Greenblatt, (ed.) *Meeting the Needs of People with Vision Loss: A Multidisciplinary Perspective,* Lexington, MA: *Resources for Rehabilitation*

Jim has mild athetoid cerebral palsy. He is 54, lives independently, and holds a full-time job in a bank loan department. His slurred speech and difficulty walking have never been big problems, although he does many things more slowly than other people. Jim is having difficulty reading reports and computer documents. There never seems to be enough light, and the reading glasses he bought at the drug store don't help at all. He is also having more trouble than usual communicating, especially over the phone. Jim thought his co-workers were used to his speech, but lately he seems to be getting a lot of funny looks, almost as though there was something wrong with what he said rather than how he said it. Jim is getting worried; he does not understand what is happening. He is much too young to retire, but work has become so stressful that he is thinking about quitting.

These scenarios describe what life can be like for older adults who are experiencing vision and hearing problems. Like the majority of people with vision and hearing impairments, their losses are age-related. The sensory losses that they are experiencing are affecting their ability to maintain their independence and quality of life.

Definitions

In order to provide services that can improve the quality of life and independence of older adults, it is important to understand vision and hearing impairments.

The "legal" definition of blindness, developed to determine eligibility for services from government programs, is an acuity of 20/200 or less in the better eye with the best possible correction or a visual field of 20 degrees or less. Most people who are legally blind, perhaps as many as 85%, have some useful vision (Jose: 1983; Hiatt: 1980). Difficulty reading newspaper print is often used as another definition of visual impairment (Branch et al.: 1989). Some individuals are not legally blind, yet have difficulty with visual tasks. These people have useful vision and are able to perform some visual tasks but are limited in performing others. The extent to which residual vision is useful depends upon a number of factors including environmental conditions, other sensory losses, other chronic conditions, and access to rehabilitation services.

Defining hearing impairment is much more difficult, since there is no "legal" definition. Most definitions used to determine eligibility for educational or rehabilitation programs focus on how hearing loss affects the ability to use language and speech.

There are some generally accepted guidelines for defining hearing impairment (Knauf: 1978). A profound hearing loss or deafness is the inability to hear any sound below 91 decibels in the better ear. A severe hearing loss is defined as the inability to hear sound below 71 decibels. People with a severe hearing loss typically have a great deal of difficulty comprehending speech and are often considered deaf. An individual with a moderately severe hearing loss cannot hear sounds below 56 decibels. A moderate hearing loss is the inability to hear sounds below 41 decibels, while a person with a mild loss cannot hear sounds below 26 decibels (Knauf: 1978; McFarland and Cox: 1987).

The ability to use remaining hearing depends on many factors. A major consideration is the frequency of the sounds associated with the loss, especially in the cases of mild to moderate loss. Effective use of remaining hearing is also influenced by environmental conditions, other sensory losses, other chronic health conditions, and the access to rehabilitation and audiological services.

When using these definitions of vision or hearing loss, it is important to remember that quantitative measurements of acuity do not take into consideration the other factors that affect a person's ability to cope with and adapt to a sensory loss. Nor do they reflect environmental factors that are beyond the individual's control. Objective measures of vision and hearing cannot be used to predict independence or functional abilities because of the variability in each individual's reaction to sensory losses.

The combined loss of vision and hearing is overwhelming and frightening to many people. The impact of these two sensory losses has much more than a simple additive effect (Luey et al.: 1989). This dual loss makes many of the adaptive techniques developed for either vision or hearing loss unusable without extensive and painstaking modification. Adaptive techniques developed for blind people rely heavily on hearing, while those for deaf people rely on vision. A dual loss forces the individual to use tactile adaptations. Such adaptations are extremely time consuming and require a great deal of concentration, stamina, and motivation.

Etiology

Older adults face two problems with their vision and hearing: normal age-related vision and hearing changes (known as presbyopia and presbycusis) and abnormal age-related disorders. Because these conditions vary in degree, the difference between normal and abnormal "changes or losses" can be arbitrary, making functional criteria for determining disability critical.

The age-related vision changes that are considered normal include increased sensitivity to glare, increased need for light, slower distance accommodation, slower adjustment to different light conditions, reduced contrast sensitivity, and reduced hue discrimination (Owsley and Sloane: 1990; Morse et al.: 1987). These normal vision changes may cause significant problems with everyday activities, particularly when they are combined with another sensory loss or chronic condition. The leading causes of new blindness among older adults are cataract, age-related macular degeneration, diabetic retinopathy, and glaucoma (National Society to Prevent Blindness, 1980). Cataracts, which are opacities of the lens, are related to the changes in the lens that cause problems with glare and accommodation. There is a similar link between changes in the retina that cause reduced contrast sensitivity and hue discrimination and age-related macular degeneration (Owsley and Sloane: 1990).

Presbycusis refers to changes in hearing caused by aging and affected by heredity, diet, and environment (Hull: 1978). Presbycusis is generally sensorineural, involving the nerves of the inner ear. Speech discrimination is reduced, especially in environments that are noisy or that have poor acoustics, and speech is distorted, regardless of its volume. Higher frequency sounds, such as "th" and "f" cannot be heard. The most difficult problem facing the older adult with age-related hearing loss is not the loss of acuity or sensitivity to sound, but problems with speech discrimination (Cox and McFarland: 1987). The ability to hear high frequency sounds and consonants is also affected. An individual may have a mild loss of sensitivity to sound but have a severe problem discriminating speech. The result is the common complaint, "I can hear you, but I cannot understand you."

The medical conditions that place older adults at risk for hearing loss include vascular disease, metabolic diseases, and infections. Several of the drugs commonly used by older adults are toxic to the auditory system. Ototoxicity should always be investigated whenever an older adult is experiencing hearing problems. Tinnitus, a ringing, buzzing, or noise in the ear, is another problem frequently encountered by older adults; it is a symptom rather than a disease and has many causes including cardiovascular disorders, head trauma, medications (particularly aspirin, tobacco, and caffeine), and accumulated noise damage (Schleuning: 1989; Vernon: 1989).

An older adult who is experiencing vision loss in conjunction with a hearing loss may also have difficulty maintaining spatial orientation. Vision and the kinesthetic system also contribute to the maintenance of equilibrium (Goeyzinger: 1978), as does the vestibular system. Many of the diseases that affect hearing also affect this system.

Demographics

Unfortunately, it is impossible to give an exact number or even an estimate of the number of older adults with both vision and hearing losses. By the year 2030, one out of every four Americans will be over 65 (U.S. Senate Select Committee on Aging: 1985). This projection, coupled with statistics on vision loss and hearing loss, suggest that there will be a large increase in the number of older Americans with impaired vision and hearing.

The incidence and prevalence of both vision and hearing impairments increase with age (National Resource Center on Health Promotion and Aging: 1990; Glass: 1983; National Society to Prevent Blindness: 1980). Vision and hearing impairments are both among the most common physical impairments of people over the age of 65. Estimates vary: however, there may be as many as ten million older adults who have a hearing impairment (National Institute on Aging: 1983). Estimates also indicate that the number of visually impaired older adults will roughly equal those experiencing Alzheimer's disease (Crews: 1988). According to the one study which provides an indication of the number of individuals who have the most severe vision and hearing impairments (Wolfe et al.: 1982), the prevalence of deaf-blindness increases with age.

The growing incidence of vision and hearing impairments, separately and in combination, as well as the aging of the general population, has major implications for health and rehabilitation professionals and caretakers, whether professional, volunteer, or family members.

Service Needs

Susan needs independent living and rehabilitation services in order to maintain her independence. Her family needs to understand what Susan is capable of doing and how they can provide appropriate assistance.

Linda's behavior is related to her sensory losses and the inability to receive information from her environment. She and the nursing home staff need a communication system. Linda also needs activities that will keep her in touch with the world around her.

Mary needs comprehensive vision and hearing testing to determine if her behavior problems are the result of presbyopia and presbycusis. If Mary has significant vision and hearing losses, staff will need to identify ways to make her environment more structured and adapt their communication techniques.

Jim also needs comprehensive vision and hearing testing. He needs to learn how to adapt his environment and develop new techniques for his work and home situations.

Recognizing an older adult's sensory losses is the first step in providing appropriate services. Vision and hearing losses are viewed by many health care professionals and older adults as an inevitable part of growing older (Weinstein: 1989; Branch et al.: 1989). The extension of that belief is that there is nothing that can be done, regardless of the severity of the loss. Because these conditions cannot be cured medically, physicians often give their older patients a "nothing can be done" prognosis (Silverstone: 1990). Regardless of the age of onset, individuals with disabilities, such as Susan, Linda, Mary, and Jim, can benefit from rehabilitation services. Too often a decline in an older adult's ability to function independently is misunderstood. Professional service providers often apply labels that denote cognitive impairment such as dementia, senility, and even Alzheimer's disease. Vision and hearing assessments should be automatic when behavioral or functional changes occur (Bagley: 1989). On the other hand, when vision and hearing losses are identified, it cannot be assumed that there are no other physical and cognitive losses. Whether or not a specific vision or hearing loss is considered disabling, rehabilitation services exist which may enable older adults to maintain or improve their independence and quality of life.

Once the individual's sensory loss or losses are diagnosed, there must be appropriate referral for rehabilitation services. In order to make appropriate referrals, professionals must understand their own and other service delivery systems. Too often professionals who encounter older adults become so involved in the specific problem that brought the individual to their attention (e.g., a vision impairment or the need for nursing care) that other problems are not recognized or addressed. Sensitivity to the constellation of problems which complicate the individual's primary service need is critical.

Rehabilitation instruction has positive effects on functioning, anxiety, and self-esteem of older blind adults (Hensley: 1987), and also relieves stress on their families (Crews and Frey: 1988). The specific services needed by older adults with age-related sensory losses vary, depending on individual situations. There are, however, at least three critical service areas to consider: communication, transportation, and community/program integration.

Transportation and community integration are closely related. Without transportation services, older adults are not able to go to community services sites, such as senior centers, medical clinics, nutrition programs, or social activities. Once they are able to attend these programs, they have the added problem of integration. How can they become a part of activities when they have difficulty seeing and hearing? No matter how transportation problems are solved, communication is the most difficult problem faced by older adults with sensory losses and their caregivers. An individual with vision and hearing impairments loses the ability to receive information from the environment, such as messages from other individuals, warning signals, and the everyday background sounds and sights that keep people in touch with their surroundings.

A tactile sign language is the communication method most frequently associated with severe deaf-blindness. There are, however, a number of other methods that build on past experience and offer a more accessible method of communication (Arkansas Rehabilitation Research and Training Center: 1984). Block printing on the palm, alphabet gloves, and raised block letters can be utilized by anyone who can read. The American one-hand or manual alphabet, which utilizes a hand symbol for each letter, can be taught and used tactually. Morse code and braille can be used on the hand, arm, or back. A limited number of survival signs can also be taught in order to speed up the communication process (see Arkansas Rehabilitation Research and Training Center: 1984 for a comprehensive overview of these methods).

Assistive listening devices enhance auditory communication by compensating for competing background noise, distance, or room echo. The four main types of assistive listening devices are infrared, induction loop, FM, and hard-wired systems (see Compton and Brandt: 1987 for a description of these devices).

Individuals use limited vision more effectively with a wide variety of low vision aids, including magnifiers, telescopes, closed circuit television systems, and lighting and color contrast techniques.

Rehabilitation professionals who work with deaf-blind adults are aware of these communication techniques and devices, as well as a wide range of coping strategies, mobility techniques, assistive aids, and techniques of daily living. These techniques and devices are largely unavailable to older adults because the health care, rehabilitation, and aging networks are not adequately linked. Many professionals within the aging network are not aware of these services. Many rehabilitation professionals who focus on one disability are unaware of the adaptations developed to deal with dual disabilities.

Older adults with sensory losses also need medical and social support services. The required medical support services range from routine screening and accurate information to prescription of assistive devices and surgery. Older adults and those who work with them need accurate, comprehensible medical information, as well as referral information and treatment and rehabilitation options.

Social supports also play a critical role for older adults with sensory losses. Formal and informal support groups, self-help groups, peer counselors, and social organizations provide social support for older adults. Support groups created through national or local organizations to assist people with special "problems" have a long history. Peer counseling has been a very successful mechanism for providing support to people in situations that are unfamiliar and threatening. Peer counseling occurs between people who understand each other because of common experience, such as age and sensory impairment. Many older adults have extremely negative feelings about vision and hearing losses and about the service systems designed to assist people with these losses (Byers-Lang: 1984). Peer counselors are especially helpful in this situation and are an important part of the service team, for they share the personal effects of sensory loss.

Support or self-help groups provide important information about sensory loss and coping strategies, as well as opportunities for socializing and combating the isolation so often experienced by older adults with sensory losses. Formal and informal support groups provide an important mechanism to keep the older adult with sensory impairments linked to the community. Numerous support/self-help groups exist for visually impaired adults (Weisse: 1989). These groups are often associated with independent living programs for older adults who are visually impaired, lighthouses for the blind, low vision clinics, or other private organizations. Self Help for Hard of Hearing People, Inc. and the Association of Late Deafened Adults are two national support organizations with local chapters for hearing impaired adults (Resources for Rehabilitation: 1990).

Unfortunately, older adults with both vision and hearing losses often find participation in single disability groups difficult and frustrating. Groups designed for people with vision impairments use auditory communication techniques, while those for people who are hearing impaired rely heavily on visual communication. Specialized groups or special sensitivity to the combination of sensory losses is important in making support services accessible to older adults with dual sensory impairments.

Formal counseling services are important to both older adults and their families. Professional assistance is often required to facilitate the adjustment process and to learn coping strategies. Assertiveness and self-advocacy training are also important services that can be provided through counseling.

There are many older adults with vision and hearing impairments who have additional specialized needs. People with disabilities acquired at birth, during childhood, or middle age also acquire age-related sensory impairments. In the past, people with severe congenital disabilities had short life expectancies, while many people did not survive disabling trauma. Advanced medical treatment has made it possible for severely disabled people to survive disabling trauma and to live many years beyond that trauma. The acquisition of age-related sensory losses complicates their adaptation and requires further rehabilitation service. Adjusted levels of support may be necessary in order to maintain independence, particularly for individuals who are multiply disabled and severely developmentally disabled.

Service Delivery

Susan's ophthalmologist referred her to an independent living program for elders with vision impairments, where she received rehabilitation teaching and mobility services. Her family also learned ways to assist Susan. A volunteer now visits her twice a week, relieving the family of some responsibilities and providing Susan with social support.

Linda now lives in a group home for people who are deaf-blind, where the staff have taught her to use a receptive communication system. The social worker at the nursing home where she formerly lived contacted a long term care ombudsman, who in turn contacted a teacher at the local rehabilitation agency. All three professionals assisted in Linda's move to the group home.

Mary received comprehensive hearing testing from an audiologist and vision testing from an optometrist skilled in testing individuals who are developmentally disabled. They referred the staff from Mary's residential institution to a national organization providing services for individuals with vision and hearing impairments. Linkages were developed with local rehabilitation programs, and the staff received special training to help them effectively communicate and plan an appropriate program for Mary.

Jim's ophthalmologist identified several visual problems and referred him to a low vision specialist. The low vision specialist helped Jim develop more effective strategies for reading and writing and referred him to a university audiology program, where he received a hearing test and learned to use assistive listening devices.

The benefits Susan, Linda, Mary, and Jim derived from the services they received depended in large part on how the services were provided. Many rehabilitation professionals encounter problems when working with older adults. These problems stem not from their skills or techniques, but the way in which they approach older clients. Older adults do not see rehabilitation services as an investment in their future but as a method to solve today's problems. They are not willing to participate in comprehensive rehabilitation service plans that take many months to complete.

Goals set by older adults are more individualistic, time limited, and focused on specific activities than those of younger people. Professionals working with older adults must recognize that the client is free to make choices and must value the small successes or "small gains" resulting from these very specific choices (Silverstone: 1984; Williams: 1984; Crews: 1988). Service delivery should focus on interdependence, which implies a mix of independence and dependence. As Katz and associates (1983) noted, rather than death, "the end point of life expectancy is the loss of independence in the activities of daily living." The quality of life will remain higher if the individual is able to retain independence in as many areas of daily life as possible.

Acceptance of rehabilitation services also depends upon the environment in which they are provided. Rehabilitation services focused on solving specific problems - crossing the street, hearing the doorbell, or independent grooming - are most quickly and effectively solved in the individual's home environment.

Although provision of rehabilitation services at a residential center is common, this setting is not effective for everyone. For older adults, the stress of adjusting to a foreign environment makes the generalization of new skills to the home situation very difficult. In addition, "institutionalization" can be very disconcerting for someone who has lived independently for 40 to 50 years.

Appropriate rehabilitative and support services will make it possible for some residents of nursing homes to regain their independence. The more likely scenario is that appropriate rehabilitation services will buy time for the older adult with sensory losses to remain connected to the community, to enjoy life, and to maintain what has been gained throughout life. As services are designed and delivered, it is important to recognize "that each task, no matter how small, creates dignity and provides the enfranchisement of independence" (Crews: 1988).

Older adults who have both vision and hearing losses need a continuum of opportunity. They must be able to choose levels of support and independence appropriate to their unique situations rather than be forced to make all or nothing choices. They must have access to services that are flexible enough to meet their specific needs. There must be flexibility in goal setting, location of service provision, and values placed on outcomes.

Service Linkages

Silverstone (1990) asserts, "No condition incurred by an older person can be treated in isolation." Hence the need for a multidisciplinary approach to the delivery of services to all older adults, and particularly those with both vision and hearing impairments.

Multidisciplinary team members should be drawn from the systems providing services needed by older adults with sensory impairments: health care, rehabilitation, and the aging network. Although the members of the multidisciplinary team may change, such an approach must be used throughout the service delivery process. It is important to establish core team members. Although each member may not always play an active role in the service delivery, their support will facilitate the effectiveness of the team. Physicians and nonprofessional caregivers such as spouses, children, grandchildren, and close friends will contribute significantly to the success of rehabilitation services through their cooperation and support.

Health care professionals who provide services needed by older adults with sensory losses can be found in private practice, medical clinics, public health organizations, acute care facilities (such as hospitals), and long term care facilities (such as nursing homes). They include, but are not limited to geriatricians, medical internists, otologists, ophthalmologists, optometrists, nurses, nurse practitioners, nurses aides, and home health aides.

Rehabilitation professionals are located in a variety of settings including state rehabilitation agencies, independent living centers, rehabilitation facilities (public and private), and private practice. Those professionals with the skills necessary to meet the needs of older adults with vision and hearing impairments work in programs specializing in services for people who are visually impaired or blind, hearing impaired or deaf, or deaf-blind. They include, but are not limited to, rehabilitation teachers, orientation and mobility instructors, occupational therapists, physical therapists, counselors, low vision specialists, rehabilitative audiologists, assistive listening device specialists, and speech pathologists.

Aging network professionals are located in a wide variety of community service settings which receive federal funding through contracts with Area Agencies on Aging and State Units on Aging. Important service providers from the aging network include, but are not limited to social workers, long term care advocates, nutrition specialists, gerontologists, senior center coordinators, nutrition site supervisors, volunteers, in-home companions, and volunteer program coordinators.

Although there is some overlap between these service systems, each operates separately and has its own goals and funding sources. The professionals listed can often be found within any of the three service systems. The professionals of greatest value to the team will have a multidisciplinary perspective and a broad understanding of the service needs of older adults, regardless of the service setting.

Independent living programs are a mechanism through which services for older adults may best be provided. Unfortunately, the scope of services provided by most centers for independent living (CIL) is limited by a lack of funding, making it difficult for them to provide comprehensive services to everyone in need. As long as CILs continue to see employment issues as the most serious problem they face (Mathews: 1989), they will not be able to adequately serve the large number of older adults with sensory impairments who need rehabilitation and support services to remain independent.

Although there appears to be little information sharing between Area Agencies on Aging (AAA) and centers for independent living, professionals in both settings have positive attitudes toward opportunities for increased interaction (Mathews: 1989). The major barriers to interaction between AAAs and rehabilitation agencies are unclear and differing expectations (Biegel et al. 1989). The linkage between the systems must be strengthened in order for multidisciplinary teams to work effectively.

Positive working relationships can only be developed if professionals within each system clearly understand what each has to offer to the older adult with sensory impairments. They must be able to look beyond their particular area of expertise to identify all of the problems experienced by the older adult and the possible solutions to those problems. The ability to work cooperatively is critical to development of multidisciplinary teams and linking service systems.

To be effective, leaders of multidisciplinary teams must keep team members informed and monitor the progress of the sensory impaired older adult. The case manager keeps the team clearly focused on the individual's changing needs. Ideally, older adults with sensory impairments would act as their own case managers. Too often, unfamiliarity with service systems, negative attitudes about services, and other chronic conditions make this impossible. Many older adults find self-advocacy and questioning of perceived authority difficult. They must be active participants in the team's planning and goal setting to the extent possible.

84

The multidisciplinary service delivery team will have a number of tasks such as development of goals, service coordination, and advocacy. The way these tasks are performed will depend upon the information available to the team. The team must also develop a system for organizing the medical, functional, and social information gathered in the course of providing services.

Without critically analyzing and organizing client data, the service delivery team risks making inappropriate decisions based upon data that are incomplete, inaccurate, or overlooked. It is important to understand what questions to ask, who to ask them of, and how to resolve apparent conflicts in available information. Too often service providers accept information that is not accurate or that they do not understand because they do not feel comfortable questioning physicians or family members. Unfortunately, many of the people providing client information do not know what the team really needs to know. The team must learn to ask the right questions of reliable information sources.

Conclusions

Achieving the goal of independence for older adults with sensory losses requires that service providers and older adults stop accepting vision and hearing impairments as an inevitable part of the aging process. Federal, state, and local governments must make a commitment to meeting the needs of older adults with vision and hearing losses. Programs and change must occur in three areas: research, model service delivery, and social attitudes.

Research, particularly in the area of demographics, is critical. Program planners must know how many older adults have vision and hearing losses that affect the routine activities of daily living. Accurate statistics are necessary to prevent inaccurate estimates of service needs and development of unnecessary services or worse yet, development of a service model inadequate to meet the need.

Demographic research will also provide information about the characteristics of older adults with dual sensory impairments. How many of these individuals live in the community versus long term care facilities? Do they have a common constellation of age-related chronic conditions that will affect service provision? And what resources are currently available to these people to meet the challenge of sensory impairments? Answers to questions such as these will allow planners to develop programs with appropriate components, in locations of greatest need, and with adequate financial and community support.

Research to develop adaptive equipment to specifically meet the needs of people with vision and hearing losses is critically needed. Some adaptations have been made to existing equipment originally designed for people who are blind or deaf. Unfortunately, this leads to adaptations that are often cumbersome and awkward. Because of limited resources, these adaptations are often not readily reproducible.

Model service delivery programs must be established to serve as guides for the development of a comprehensive service system designed to meet the needs of older adults with vision and hearing losses. These model programs must include prevention of sensory impairments; a holistic approach to service delivery; linkage of existing service delivery systems; expanding the service delivery team; and professional personnel preparation.

Model programs must include a public education component focused on prevention. The impact of vision and hearing losses encountered by older adults can be reduced through regular ophthalmological exams, compliance with medical advice, and protecting the ears from excessive environmental noise (Bagley: 1989).

Model programs and the professionals working within them must take a holistic approach to service delivery. Rehabilitation providers tend to focus on specific problems, while specialists providing services to older adults tend to be too global. As Silverstone (1990) points out, this is due in part to the categorical way services are organized and funded. Team members must be able to look at specific problems within the overall context of the person's situation.

Strong linkages must be made between all of the providers of services to older adults. Rehabilitation professionals must become an integral link in that chain of services. Once health care, rehabilitation, and aging network programs become linked, those linkages must be nurtured in order to achieve a holistic approach without losing the specific skills offered by each professional (Silverstone: 1990).

Multidisciplinary training during the personnel preparation process will help to promote understanding, foster the development of multi-disciplinary teams, and promote agency linkages. Not only must rehabilitation professionals who specialize in vision and hearing impairments learn about aging, but specialists in aging services must learn about sensory rehabilitation. It is not enough for rehabilitation professionals to learn techniques that they will have to adjust for older people. They must learn why older adults require a different approach to services and what that approach is. Vision specialists must learn about hearing impairment, and specialists in deafness must also learn about vision impairment. Health care professionals need to learn about rehabilitation and its potential to help the person for whom they can provide no further medical help.

Social change is the final and perhaps most important requirement in the quest to achieve independence for older adults with vision and hearing impairments. Health care, rehabilitation, and aging network professionals must recognize the functional effects of a disability and the associated need for intervention regardless of age. Society must not allow the loss of independence resulting from sensory impairments to be an acceptable part of aging. Older adults must not lose their independence and quality of life because rehabilitation services are focused on younger people. Health and rehabilitation professionals as well as professionals in the field of aging must reaffirm the innate dignity of the individual and make a commitment to the individual's right to independence.

References

Arkansas Rehabilitation Research and Training Center in Vocational Rehabilitation
1984   *Strategies for Serving Deaf-Blind Clients: Eleventh Institute of Rehabilitation Issues* Hot Springs, AR: University of Arkansas

Bagley, Martha
1989   *Identifying Vision and Hearing Problems Among Older Persons: Strategies and Resources*   Sands Point, NY: Helen Keller National Center for Deaf-Blind Youths and Adults

Biegel, David E., Marcia K. Petchers, Arlene Snyder, and Beverly Beisgen
1989   "Unmet Needs and Barriers to Service Delivery for the Blind and Visually Impaired Elderly" *The Gerontologist* 29(1):86

Branch, Laurence G., Amy Horowitz, and Cheryl Carr
1989   "The Implications for Everyday Life of Incident Self-Reported Visual Decline Among People Over 65 Living in the Community" *The Gerontologist* 29(3):359-365

Byers-Lang, Rosalind
1984   "Peer Counselors: Network Builders for Elderly Persons" *Journal of Visual Impairment and Blindness* 78(5):193-197

Compton, Cynthia L. and Fred D. Brandt
1987   *Assistive Listening Devices: A Consumer-Oriented Summary* Washington, DC: Gallaudet University

Cox, B. Patrick and William H. McFarland
1987   "Audiologic Aspects of Aging" pp. 8-15 in Maureen Durkin (ed.) *When Hearing Fades* Washington, DC: Gallaudet University Press

Crews, John E.
1988   "No One Left To Push: The Public Policy of Aging and Blindness" *Educational Gerontology* 14(5):399-409

Crews, John E. and William Frey
1988   "Family Stress and Older Blind Persons: An Examination of the Concerns of Caregivers With Older Blind Family Members" Paper presented at *Age-related Vision Loss: Development in Low Vision Practices and Research* Symposium marking the 35th anniversary of the Lighthouse, Inc., New York, NY

Glass, Laurel
1983   "Psychological Aspects of Hearing Loss in Adulthood" H. Orlans (ed.) *Adjustment to Adult Hearing Loss* San Diego, CA: College Hill Press

Goeyzinger, Cornelius D.
1978   "The Psychology of Hearing Impairment" p. 459 in Jack Katz (ed.) *Handbook of Clinical Audiology* Baltimore, MD: Williams and Wilkins

Hensley, Mike
1987   "Rehabilitation in Daily Living Skills: Effects On Anxiety and Self-Worth in Elderly Blind Persons" *Journal of Visual Impairment and Blindness* 81(7):330

Hiatt, Lorraine
1980   "Is Poor Light Dimming the Sight of Nursing Home Patients?" *Nursing Homes* 29(5):32-41

Hull, Raymond
1978   "Hearing Evaluation of the Elderly" p. 416 in Jack Katz (ed.) *Handbook of Clinical Audiology* Baltimore, MD: Williams and Wilkins

Jose, Randall
1983   "The Low Vision Rehabilitation Service" pp. 61-71 in Randall Jose (ed.) *Understanding Low Vision* New York, NY: American Foundation for the Blind

Katz, S., L.G. Branch, M.H. Branson, J.A. Papsidero, J.C. Beck, and D.S. Greer
1983   "Active Life Expectancy" *New England Journal of Medicine* 369(20):1218-1224

Knauf, Vincent H.
1978   "Language and Speech Training" pp. 549-564 in Jack Katz (ed.) *Handbook of Clinical Audiology* Baltimore, MD: Williams and Wilkins

Luey, Helen, Dmitri Belser, and Laurel Glass
1989   *Beyond Refuge: Coping with Losses of Vision and Hearing in Later Life* Sands Point, NY: Helen Keller National Center for Deaf-Blind Youths and Adults

Mathews, R. Mark
1989   *Switzer Fellowship Field Report* Unpublished manuscript

McFarland, William, and Patrick B. Cox
1987   *Aging and Hearing Loss: Some Commonly Asked Questions* Washington, DC: Gallaudet University Press

Morse, Alan R., Roseann Silberman, and Ellen Trief
1987   "Aging and Visual Impairment" *Journal of Visual Impairment and Blindness* 81(7):308-312

National Institute on Aging
1983   *Age Page: Hearing and the Elderly* Washington, DC: U.S. Government Printing Office

National Resource Center on Health Promotion and Aging
1990   *Perspectives* 5(3)

National Society to Prevent Blindness
1980   *Vision Problems in the U.S.* New York, NY: National Society to Prevent Blindness

Owsley, Cynthia and Michael Sloane
1990   "Vision and Aging" pp. 229-249 in F. Boller and J. Grafman (eds.) *Handbook of Neuropsychology* *Volume 4* Elsevier Science Publishers B.V.

Resources for Rehabilitation
1990   *Resources for Elders with Disabilities* Lexington, MA: Resources for Rehabilitation

Schleuning, Alexander
1989   "Medical Aspects of Tinnitus" *The Hearing Journal* 43(11):12-15

Select Committee on Aging
1985   *Hearing on Blindness and the Elderly* House of Representatives
        Ninety-ninth Congress, First Session Publication No. 99-519
        Washington, DC: U.S. Government Printing Office

Silverstone, Barbara
1990   "Setting an Agenda for the Future" Paper presented at *The
        Challenge to Independence: Vision and Hearing Loss Among
        Older Adults* Dallas, TX
1984   "Social Aspects of Rehabilitation" pp.59-80 in T. Franklin
        Williams (ed.) *Rehabilitation in Aging* New York, NY: Raven
        Press

Vernon, Jack
1989   "Tinnitus 1989: Current Knowledge and Treatment Therapy"
        The Hearing Journal 42(11):7-11

Weinstein, Barbara E.
1989   "Geriatric Hearing Loss: Myths, Realities, Resources for Physi-
        cians" *Geriatrics* 44(4):42-59

Weisse, Fran A.
1989   "Self-Help Groups for People with Vision Loss" pp. 84-99 in
        Susan L. Greenblatt (ed.) *Providing Services for People with
        Vision Loss: A Multidisciplinary Perspective* Lexington, MA:
        Resources for Rehabilitation

Williams, T. Franklin
1984   *Rehabilitation in the Aging* New York, NY: Raven Press

Wolfe, Enid, Marcus Delk, and Jerome Schein
1982   *Needs Assessment of Services to Deaf-Blind Individuals* Silver
        Spring, MD: Rehabilitation and Education Experts, Inc.

*   Special credit must be given to John Mascia, Coordinator of
        Audiological Services at the Helen Keller National Center, for his
        advice, support, and review of this document. Dennis Brady,
        Assistant Director of the Helen Keller National Center, also
        provided critical comments that have contributed to this chapter.

Providing Services To Visually Impaired Elders In Long Term Care Facilities: A Multidisciplinary Approach

Maureen A. Duffy, M.S.
Monica Beliveau-Tobey, M.Ed.

Consider the following demographic trends:

• The population age 65 and older is projected to grow to 52 million by 2020; this represents an increase of 75% over 1987 figures. By 2030, the elderly population should be at least 59 million, or double its present size (Spencer: 1989).

• The number of individuals age 85 and older will approximately double during the next 20 years (Spencer: 1989).

• Approximately 80% of persons over the age of 75 are likely to experience some degree of functional visual disability (Fozard and Popkin: 1978) which can significantly affect the maintenance of independent living skills.

• Lowman and Kirchner (1979) and Kirchner and Peterson (1979) report that demographic patterns clearly isolate *age* as the single most powerful predictor of blindness and visual impairment.

According to Wineburg, most visually impaired elders:

...are newly blind, have some remaining vision, are mainly over 75 years of age, and are usually poor...They are most

Susan L. Greenblatt, (ed.) Meeting the Needs of People with Vision Loss: A Multidisciplinary Perspective, Lexington, MA: Resources for Rehabilitation often people who have become blind at a late age, when they are also dealing with other physiological, psychological, and social problems which also accompany aging. (1981, p. 58)

Nelson reports an updated analysis of data from the National Center for Health Statistics (NCHS), indicating that "the prevalence of visual impairment among elderly people is much higher than previously supposed," due to refinements in NCHS's research methods (1987, p. 334). Comparison of 1984 data to 1977 data shows an increase of 106% in the number of persons 65 or over who are visually impaired.

Let us now consider statistics regarding numbers of older persons in long term care facilities in conjunction with those cited above:

• The 1985 summary of *The National Nursing Home Survey* (NNHS) estimated that (a) approximately 5% of the population age 65 and older can expect to reside in a long term care facility; (b) persons age 65 and older comprised the majority (93%) of all nursing home residents; and (c) approximately 2.5% of all residents were totally blind, while another 22% were partially to severely visually impaired (Hing et al.: 1989).

• Hing and Sekscenski also note that "A change ... occurred in the age distribution of nursing home residents during the period 1977-1985, with a shift toward the oldest age groups. Whereas 35% of all residents in 1977 were 85 years of age and over, 40% of 1985 residents were in that age group." (1987, p. 71)

• It has also been estimated that over 50% of all nursing home residents "[have] vision impairments warranting intervention" (Hiatt: 1980, p. 34).

Despite identification of the high prevalence of visual impairment among residents of long term care facilities, it is likely that significant numbers of older persons in long term care remain unidentified and/or unreported. Yeadon concurs with this assessment, suggesting that "many people... living within these environments are not given appropriate diagnoses or treatment..." (1984, p. 149).

Why is it difficult to gauge the full extent of the older visually impaired population in long term care facilities? Why do reported numbers of institutionalized visually impaired elders remain low, while prevalence estimates of vision impairment in the noninstitutionalized older adult population continue to climb? Yeadon (1984) believes that a number of complex factors intertwine to cause resident/patient nondisclosure, including a sense of pride and fear of dependency or of "being a burden" (p. 149).

Byers-Lang (1984) reported that older visually impaired adults in her peer counseling program initially derived considerable group status through the process of mutual ranking according to perceived amounts of usable vision. Hiatt observed that "older people conceal vision changes, worrying that failing memories [are] the cause of problems, or fearing that they might be relocated to higher... levels of care" (1980, p. 34). Yeadon (1984), Orr (1987), and Hiatt (1980) concur that older persons may accept gradually diminishing or failing vision as a normal part of the aging process and thus may not actively seek appropriate eye care or medical intervention.

Long term care facility staff's knowledge of issues related to vision loss and the need for in-service staff training have been addressed extensively by Wineburg (1982), who forcefully advocates for the development and rigorous evaluation of in-service training programs targeted to the special needs of both staff and visually impaired residents. In Wineburg's view, appropriate staff training and timely referral for resident/patient eye care are germane:

> It is apparent that nursing home staff share the general public's misunderstanding of blindness... [and that they] lack the skills needed to aid elderly blind people's 'adequate" adjustment to the nursing home facilities... Successful in-service training on blindness would substantially aid staff in acquiring skills in detecting visual problems and teaching residents how to eat, dress, and even groom themselves. There is a good chance that nursing homes that have staffs grounded in how to work with visually impaired residents might become places where elderly people get well or have a good chance of

getting well because they get diagnosed and treated properly. (1982, pp. 70, 72)

Hiatt (1980, 1981), Morse and associates (1988), and Wineburg (1982) note, however, that several barriers to effective ongoing training continue to exist within the institutional structure, including a lack of systematic annual vision screening policies; high rates of staff turnover; differential learning capabilities of staff; facility design and layout; difficulty maintaining an interdisciplinary approach to resident care; and tenuous intersystem linkages between the blind service system and the nursing home network.

Strong demographic trends coupled with the observations of the authors cited above convinced researchers in the Department of Graduate Studies in Vision Impairment at the Pennsylvania College of Optometry (PCO) that a training curriculum targeted specifically to staff of long term care facilities could significantly improve the quality of life for residents. This chapter will discuss two research studies and a training program for service providers in long term care facilities.

A National Survey

The initial study, which assessed current practices in long term care facilities for visually impaired residents, revealed a striking dearth of staff training and knowledge (Beliveau et al.: 1986). A questionnaire was pilot-tested, revised, and sent to 2,000 randomly selected facilities listed in the 1982 National Master Facility Inventory of the National Center for Health Statistics (NCHS). The final return rate was 25.7% or 513 responses.

The majority (81.6%) of the residents in the responding long term care facilities were over 75 years, with 42.4% over the age of 85 years. Identification of residents' visual impairments was the result of staff observation (81%), self-reports (66%), and reports of family and friends (47%), rather than through required, periodic eye examinations and/or vision screenings.

Sixty-seven percent of the responding facilities had no policy on vision examinations. Four percent required a current vision examination only for those newly admitted residents known to be visually impaired, while 20% admitted the individual and performed a vision examination "as needed." Ninety-three percent of the respondents answered "yes" when asked if their staff would benefit from educational materials related to the care and needs of visually impaired residents. According to the respondents, the primary barriers to providing inservice education were limited staff time (65%); lack of relevant training materials (47%); and conflicts in staff scheduling patterns (44%).

Results of the survey were used to develop interviews with facility staff and residents. Ten facilities were visited, and individual or group interviews were conducted. Representative facility staff included nurses, nurses aides, social service workers, dietary workers, administrators, physicians, and rehabilitation specialists, including occupational, physical, and recreation therapists. All disciplines identified the following topics as highly relevant to their daily job performance: functional implications of vision impairment; "clues" or indicators of potential vision problems; orientation and sighted guide skills; and helping the residents to deal with the emotional impacts of vision impairment. Physicians and administrators, in particular, requested information about "model" programs relevant to the needs of the blind/visually impaired long term care population and specialists in the combined fields of aging and vision rehabilitation.

Despite criteria supplied by project staff to facility administrators regarding vision parameters for resident interviewees (i.e., a visual impairment affecting one or more areas of daily functioning that could not be corrected with regular eyeglasses alone), candidates proposed for resident interviews ranged from normally sighted (usually with glasses) to totally blind since birth. This finding supports Wineburg's (1982) assertion that many facilities do not know how to identify visually impaired residents. Problems for both the facility staff and the research team in securing accurate vision data were attributed to the lack of records of recent eye exams in medical charts; policies which protected resident confidentiality by limiting access by nonemployees (including PCO research staff) to medical charts; and notations in medical charts conflicting with residents' own statements of visual function. In addition, a quarter of the residents interviewed who had been labelled as "totally blind" actually demonstrated useful, functional vision.

Resident interview data were largely qualitative. Representative comments noted below suggest that basic rehabilitation services for visually impaired elders in nursing homes are not provided:

> I wish they could teach me how to walk safely alone.

> I hate having to wait for help with dressing [and] bathing.

> ... no one really understands what it's like to be old and almost blind.

> [I] wish some of these people would ask me what I can do, can't do, [and] how much I would like to learn to do...

These remarks also suggest that in-service training programs must be responsive to the holistic needs of visually impaired elders in long term care facilities.

Following interviews with staff and residents, an in-service workshop for educators was conducted jointly with the New York In-Service Directors' Educational Association, a professional group representing numerous long term care facilities of different sizes, types, and locations. The purpose of the workshop was to explore the specific problems inherent in the provision of in-service training in the long term care setting. The workshop participants recommended that the curriculum be flexible; include simulation, case-study activities, and self-directed learning; that each segment not exceed one hour; and that certified nursing assistants be included. It was also recommended that the curriculum be in the form of a kit consisting of workbooks, vision simulators, and resource guides, and that the kit be organized so that a wide variety of staff members would find either the whole kit or parts of it relevant and useful.

Curriculum Development

In response to the extensive needs determined by the survey described above, a project was designed to develop, field-test, produce and disseminate a self-directed, competency-based in-service curriculum package for use in long term care facilities. Following a field-test of the pilot curriculum, a complete package would be disseminated for utilization by long term care facility staff. The pilot curriculum, entitled *New Independence: Caring for the Older Visually Impaired Resident* (Duffy and Beliveau-Tobey: in press) was designed with several interrelated components: a *Learner Workbook*, containing generic knowledge/competencies; a *Facilitator/Educators Guide*, containing detailed instructions for implementing the curriculum; a set of four individual vision "distorters" provided for each learner, a *Further Learning Activities and Resources* manual, containing more advanced and discipline-specific knowledge; and a 20 minute videotape, detailing specific types of age-related vision loss, with an emphasis upon functional disability.

A wide variety of professionals contributed to the core knowledge and competencies in the curriculum. This multidisciplinary collaboration included nurses, dieticians, gerontologists, optometrists, occupational and recreation therapists, orientation and mobility specialists, rehabilitation teachers, vision rehabilitation specialists, and specialists in reading/literacy.

The pilot curriculum was field-tested in 36 randomly selected long term care facilities in Florida. Each learner group in each of the 36 nursing homes was headed by a "facilitator." A facilitator was the "team leader" who selected the five learners; distributed the study materials; administered questionnaires, pretests and posttests, and review quizzes; and supervised the entire learning process through completion. In 86% of the facilities that completed the field-test project, facilitators were also learners themselves. These individuals filled out the evaluation materials appropriate for learners, in addition to those specific to facilitators.

The sample sites were randomly assigned to three groups, with five participants from each site in each group.

1. *Trainer-Assisted*

With the cooperation of the Florida State Division of Blind Services and the Pinellas Center for the Visually Impaired (PCVI), a two-day curriculum workshop was conducted with the 12 designated facilitators/educators from each facility/site in this group. The workshop was conducted by the senior editor of the curriculum, who was also the project field-test coordinator. Disciplines represented in this group (as well as in the other two groups) included occupational and physical therapists, social workers, nurses, and staff development specialists. Participants were not informed, however, of their participation in a larger research project.

Also attending were two designated local "field-test coordinators" whose function was to provide ongoing guidelines and telephone support to the 12 trainer-assisted and 12 self-directed sites. These field-test coordinators were aware that this training was part of a research project.

2. *Self-Directed*

The sites assigned to this group tested the curriculum package independently and received no onsite consultation or support. The facilities did agree, however, to adhere to the project goals, objectives, and time lines. The designated facilitator/educator in each facility did not receive prior training in the utilization of the curriculum; instead, they were provided with an "800" telephone number which linked them to a local "field-test coordinator" who had been trained at the curriculum workshop. In addition, they also received three personal letters which encouraged them to call the toll-free telephone number if needed and reminded them to complete the evaluation materials. This system of telephone assistance most closely resembles the anticipated approach that may be offered with the final curriculum product.

3. *Control Group*

This group received no specific intervention or training. Each facility received only the curriculum package and a detailed cover letter. They were not provided with the "800" telephone number, and consequently received no guidelines or ongoing support.

All field-test participants were informed of the 12 week completion deadline, as well as the need for a minimum of five learners to complete the entire curriculum at each site.

At the completion of the 12 week field-test period, a two-day curriculum evaluation workshop was conducted by the curriculum co-editors. In attendance were the facilitators/educators from each facility that successfully completed the entire curriculum in accordance with the criteria stated above. The completion rates for the three groups were as follows: trainer-assisted, 60%; self-directed, 50%; and control, 17%. This finding suggests that some form of ongoing guidance and support is required to ensure the timely completion of the entire sequential learning process.

At the workshop, all participants praised the written materials, frequently stating that they "had never been able to find anything about blindness before." Other facilitators, primarily staff development coordinators, stated that the pilot curriculum materials would become a permanent component of all staff training packages. Although the project staff had expressed some reservations concerning the basic level of the reading materials, an occupational therapist stated that she had:

> ...finally been presented with materials about vision impairment that I can *comprehend*. Usually, I read clinical materials about blindness or the eye and just stop reading after a while, because I just don't understand, but this time I *really got it*!

This last comment should serve as a caveat to all practitioners in the vision field. It is not sufficient to speak or write (essentially to each other) in technical, jargon-laden phrases. In order to effect change and educate members of other allied health fields where practitioners encounter many elders with vision problems, simplicity of expression is a key.

In addition, most participants stated that they had minimal previous knowledge of blindness or vision impairment, and in fact, found the concepts of low vision and functional vision to be startlingly original. As one participant stated:

> I never knew that vision problems affected older people so disproportionately. We are definitely revising our estimates of the numbers of visually impaired residents in our facility.

A director of nursing stated that:

> ... I had never understood about braille before - what it was, who it would help, and who could not use it... Also, I didn't know *how* or *where* to obtain large print or recorded books. I'm going to keep and use this curriculum as a permanent resource guide.

Another director of nursing stated:

> ... it had *never* occurred to me that many residents may have been eating poorly because they couldn't *see* their food very well... The information that the curriculum provided about color, contrast, and lighting convinced me that consumption of food could be related to these factors, especially in our resident population.

All workshop participants indicated that they were eager to receive specific information that would enable them to forge linkages with appropriate agencies, services, and professionals in the blindness field. A social worker commented that:

> ... prior to this training program, I had *no idea* that there were so many different kinds of trained professionals in the "blindness" system... I had never heard of rehabilitation teachers, orientation and mobility specialists, and low vision specialists. Even if I had heard of them, I still would not have known where or whom to call for assistance.

At the conclusion of the workshop, an occupational therapist observed that the curriculum became meaningful to her nursing assistants because:

> ... it was *functional*, and not simply a collection of facts. Because nursing assistants are constantly busy attending to patient care issues, they want their in-service training to be concise and relevant. They want to be able to *help their patients*, not memorize facts.

Descriptive and statistical data obtained from the project assessment instruments support these anecdotal comments. Statistical analysis of data reported by the participants indicates that previous training in visual impairment and blindness ranged from non-existent to minimal.

On average, learners had worked with elders 7.6 years. Yet two-thirds (67%) stated that they had not received any prior education about vision and vision problems. One-third (33%) had received an average of 1.5 hours of prior training about vision and vision problems. On a scale of 0 (none) to 4 (very high), mean responses below 2.0 were recorded in response to the following knowledge self-assessment items prior to training: causes of eye disease (1.49), utilization of special low vision devices (1.66), problems caused by different eye diseases (1.70), ability to differentiate between stereotypes and facts relating to blindness (1.73), changes in the aging eye (1.81), parts of the eye (1.88), and ocular emergency signs and symptoms (1.91).

Analysis of mean pretest/posttest scores among all three groups revealed a highly significant ($p < .001$) overall training effect. The curriculum produced significant improvements in post-training knowledge regardless of level of support provided to the facilitators by the researchers.

Facilitators had worked with elders an average of 7.3 years. Nearly a quarter (23%) stated that they had not received any prior education about vision and vision problems. The remainder had received an average of 3.2 hours of prior training about vision and vision problems. Using the same scale described above for learners, the only item to receive a mean below 2.0 was utilization of special low vision devices (1.92).

Recommendations and Conclusions

Previous research has clearly indicated that large numbers of elders residing in long term care facilities may be experiencing significant functional vision impairments (Hiatt: 1980; Kirchner and Peterson: 1980; Beliveau et al.: 1986). This same research also suggests that inadequate staff training related to eye care and/or vision impairment, lack of periodic vision screenings for all residents, and a perceived lack of relevant training materials contribute to the failure to identify and rehabilitate residents with visual impairments. The research project described here suggests that a tightly focused, highly functional, multi-disciplinary in-service curriculum can remediate knowledge gaps and produce measurable gains in learner competency. The following recommendations are derived from the research findings:

- Provide learners with materials written in clear, simple language.

- Provide the curriculum in a personal workbook format, thus permitting learners to write, make notations and otherwise demonstrate personal "ownership" of the materials.

- Allow for flexibility in curriculum implementation and administration. For example, some learners may opt to utilize the materials through self-study, while others may learn best by participating in structured "traditional" classroom sessions. Still others may prefer to augment self-study with occasional participation in a facilitator-directed session. A personal workbook format permits this flexible approach.

- Break lessons/sessions into 45 minute to one-hour time periods to fit schedules in the long term care facility. Sessions can be structured so that lessons are sequential, but not neces-sarily dependent upon a fixed schedule for completion.

- Allow time for "hands-on" learning activities. In many cases, the most effective way to illustrate a functional problem caused by a particular eye disease or disorder (i.e., "tunnel vision" caused by advanced glaucoma) is by providing learners with glasses or disposable eye masks that simulate the visual effects of the condition. When used to conduct normal activities of daily living (writing, walking to the dining room, reading an activity schedule, or eating a "typical" meal), these vision "distorters" can provide skills and knowledge that are relevant to the long term care setting.

• Encourage a multidisciplinary team approach to problem solving. Many residents who are visually impaired may experience complex, overlapping disabilities, warranting input from a variety of professionals including ophthalmologists, optometrists, and rehabilitation professionals. For example, encourage nurses and assistants to study and recognize symptoms of ocular emergencies, such as retinal detachments, and to make timely, appropriate referrals to eye doctors. This is important because many eye and vision problems may occur in between regularly scheduled eye examinations or vision screenings.

Staff members in long term care facilities will adopt a "can do" attitude if provided with relevant, functional training materials. A multidisciplinary team effort will result in the accurate detection of many functional vision problems that currently go undiagnosed. Dignity and independent function will be restored for many institutionalized elders with vision loss.

References

Beliveau, Monica, Anne Yeadon, and Sheree Aston
1986   *Innovative Curriculum Development Research: To Develop In-Service Training Curriculum for Providers of Long Term Care to Elderly Blind/Visually Impaired* (Innovation Grant No. G008535147), Washington, DC: National Institute for Handicapped Research

Byers-Lang, Rosalind E.
1984   "Peer Counselors, Network Builders for Elderly Persons" *Journal of Visual Impairment and Blindness* 78(4):154-162

105

Duffy, Maureen, and Monica Beliveau-Tobey (eds.)
In press *New Independence: Caring for the Older Visually Impaired Resident*

Fozard, John L. and S. J. Popkin
1978   "Optimizing Adult Development: Ends and Means of an Applied Psychology of Aging" *American Psychologist* 33:975-989

Hiatt, Lorraine G.
1981   "The Color and Use of Color in Environments for Older People" *Nursing Homes* 30(3):8-22
1980   "Is Poor Light Dimming the Sight of Nursing Home Patients?" *Nursing Homes* 29(5):32-41

Hing, Esther, Edward Sekscenski, and Genevieve Strahan
1989   *The National Nursing Home Survey: 1985 Summary for the United States* U.S. Department of Health and Human Services, Vital and Health Statistics, Series 13, No. 97 Washington, DC: U.S. Government Printing Office

Hing, Esther and Edward Sekscenski
1987   "Use of Health Care-Nursing Home Care" p. 71 in Richard J. Havlik, Barbara Marzetta Liu, Mary Grace Kovar, Richard Suzman, Jacob J. Feldman, Tamara Harris, and Joan Van Nostrand (eds.) *Health Statistics on Older Persons, United States, 1986* U.S. Department of Health and Human Services, Vital and Health Statistics, Series 3, No. 25   Washington, DC: U.S. Government Printing Office

Kirchner, Corinne, and Richard Peterson
1979   "The Latest Data On Visual Disability from NCHS" *Journal of Visual Impairment and Blindness* 73(4):151-153

Lowman, Cherry, and Corinne Kirchner
1979   "Elderly Blind and Visually Impaired Persons: Projected Numbers in the Year 2000" *Journal of Visual Impairment and Blindness* 73(2):69-73

Morse, Alan R., William O'Connell, Joan Joseph, and Harvey Finkelstein
1988   "Assessing Vision in Nursing Home Residents" *Journal of Vision Rehabilitation* 2(4):5-14

Nelson, Katherine A.
1987   "Visual Impairment Among Elderly Americans: Statistics in Transition" *Journal of Visual Impairment and Blindness* 81(7):331-334

Orr, Alberta L.
1987   "The Elderly Visually Impaired Patient: What Every Home Care Provider Should Know" *Caring* August:55-58

Spencer, Gregory
1989   *Projections of the Population of the United States, by Age, Sex, And Race: 1988 to 2080* U.S. Bureau of the Census, Current Population Reports, Series P-25, No. 1018 Washington, DC: U.S. Government Printing Office

Wineburg, Robert J.
1982   "The Elderly Blind in Nursing Homes: The Need for a Coordinated In-Service Training Policy" *Journal of Gerontological Social Work* 4(3/4):67-77
1981   "The Elderly Blind: The Unseen" *Journal of Gerontological Social Work* 4(2):55-63

Yeadon, Anne
1984   "The Informal Care Group: Problem or Potential?" *Journal of Visual Impairment and Blindness* 78(4):149-154

Multidisciplinary Case Studies

Sarah White: A Woman
with Age-Related Macular Degeneration

Alice G. Karpik, M.D., Ophthalmologist
Barbara Davis, M.Ed., Rehabilitation Teacher

Alice G. Karpik:

Sarah White is a 76 year old woman who was first seen in 1987 and noted to have bilateral pigmented drusen in both macula. She was shown how to use an Amsler grid and asked to report any visual changes.

Fourteen months later, Mrs. White came into the clinic with vision of 20/100. She reported that for about two months she had noticed some distortion in her vision when using the Amsler grid. A fluorescein angiogram of the right eye showed a large area of neovascularization involving the fovea that could not be treated. A fluorescein angiogram of the left eye showed an area of subretinal neovascularization that did not involve the fovea, and she immediately received laser treatment.

Mrs. White's visual acuity remained at 20/100 in her right eye and 20/30 in her left eye until April, 1989. At that time, a fluorescein angiogram showed no recurrence in the area which had received laser treatment. However, when she returned one month later, there were multiple foci of recurrent subretinal neovascularization involving the fovea.

Vision remained in the 20/40 range in this eye for the next six months but dropped to 20/70 by April, 1990. By that time Mrs. White was having difficulty reading restaurant menus, writing checks, and writing her grocery list. She returned for a low vision consultation.

Susan L. Greenblatt, (ed.) Meeting the Needs of People with Vision Loss: A Multidisciplinary Perspective, Lexington, MA: Resources for Rehabilitation

Magnifiers, tinted lenses, telescopes, and loupes were tried. She took home a 6 diopter clip-on but returned it two weeks later because she had difficulty adjusting to the new working distance. She also returned the telescope but was able to use an 8X loupe and a lighted pocket magnifier. A typoscope was helpful for writing checks.

When Mrs. White was last seen in December 1990, she said that she was able to do what she wanted to do the most, read her bills and write her checks. A telescope was fitted and a closed circuit television system was demonstrated. At this time, she has little interest in any further aids, apparently because she is able to do what she wants to do.

A referral was made to a local organization which provides rehabilitation teaching services in the home to elders who are not legally blind. Their staff would assess Mrs. White's daily living skills and recommend techniques to help her use her remaining vision to its fullest potential.

Barbara Davis:

The ophthalmologist's referral states that Mrs. White has an unstable eye condition but does not include information about her visual prognosis; the existence of other eye conditions, such as cataract or glaucoma; the location of her scotomas; refractive errors/cylindrical corrections, if any; and the results of low vision testing for color, contrast, and visual fields. The referral suggests that little beyond reading problems was determined, yet one would suspect that significant loss of central vision would lead to difficulties in other areas of daily living.

It would also be helpful to know why the low vision specialist prescribed the level of magnification in these specific aids; whether it is necessary to patch the eye not being used; what type of reading materials were used with these low vision aids and what Mrs. White could read; and what recommendations were made for teaching the use of the aids.

During my first visit to Mrs. White, I asked about her functional vision. How was she using her remaining vision? Was she having difficulty in everyday tasks beyond her stated reading/writing difficulties? Had she stopped doing any activities due to vision loss?

When she offered to make me a cup of tea, I could observe how she moved about her kitchen, her pouring skills, and if she took any safety precautions while working at her stove.

We discussed the low vision aids that had been prescribed and I asked her to show me how she used them. I assessed her check-writing and bill-reading skills and considered additional aids, optical and nonoptical, which might be helpful.

I asked Mrs. White about her living situation; whether she lived alone and what type of support system of family or friends she could call on when she needed assistance. Did she use community services such as the senior center, dial-a-ride transportation, or volunteers? Does she have any health problems, such as arthritis, osteoporosis, or high blood pressure? Does she understand her visual impairment, the prognosis, and ramifications? Would she like to talk with others who have had vision loss? Is she dealing with daily activities realistically?

After the initial assessment in the home, Mrs. White and I can work together to develop a plan which will enable her to use her remaining vision most efficiently while maintaining her independence and safety in daily living. This plan may include developing efficient use of visual skills without aids, through the use of techniques such as fixation, localization, scanning and tracking; continued practice and use of prescribed optical aids; and an assessment of the lighting in her home. Nonoptical aids and techniques may be recommended, such as reading stands, bold pens, bold or raised line paper, large print reading materials, writing guides, colored filter sheets, tinted absorptive lenses, and the use of contrast and color/tactile marking materials. Training may be provided in the use of adaptive aids and/or techniques in other areas of daily living, such as personal care, home management, safety, and recreational activities. Information and resources for individuals with vision loss may also be provided.

If possible, family or significant others should be present during explanations, discussions, and training, since they often hear and remember what the individual with vision loss does not. However, if there is tension in the relationship, it is often better to work with the individual alone.

These guidelines are helpful when introducing new aids, techniques, and training. The environment should be as relaxed as possible. The individual's home is probably the most relaxed, nonthreatening environment. Initial tasks should be easy enough to ensure success, but also meaningful to the individual. Plans need to be flexible to meet the specific needs of the individual. Short instructional sessions with periods of discussion may be more comfortable for the individual.

Communication with other members of the rehabilitation team, i.e., ophthalmologist, low vision specialist, social worker, and case manager, is essential for the greatest success. In this particular case, a report of Mrs. White's home assessment, recommendations, and follow-up should be shared with the various members of the team.

Deidre Edwards:
A Child with Myopic Degeneration

Alice G. Karpik, M.D., Ophthalmologist
Susan Becker, M.Ed., Social Worker

Alice G. Karpik:

Deidre Edwards is an eight year old girl who has been referred by her optometrist for ophthalmological examination because her best corrected vision in her right eye had decreased to 20/200. Last year her vision was 20/60 in both eyes. She is wearing glasses that she has had for one year, with spherical equivalent -17.00 in the right eye, -16.00 in the left eye.

On the day of the examination, Deidre's vision was 20/50 in the right eye, 20/60 in the left eye, with best correction. Ophthalmic examination showed clear lenses and lacquer cracks in both maculas.

With her present glasses and normal room light, Deidre was able to read 12 to 14 point type. In both eyes, there was a clear central area of vision on the Amsler grid, extending for approximately 5 degrees from center of fixation, perhaps as a result of her spectacle correction.

Her parents reported that she was having difficulty with her school work. They were particularly concerned because of a strong family history of eye problems, including childhood cataract in both parents and retinal detachment in the mother and maternal grandfather.

Because her parents questioned her ability to do her school work, she returned for a low vision evaluation. Once again, she was able to

Susan L. Greenblatt, (ed.) Meeting the Needs of People with Vision Loss: A Multidisciplinary Perspective, Lexington, MA: Resources for Rehabilitation

read 12 to 14 point type in normal room light, with her glasses on, just as she had at the previous examination.

Deidre returned ten days later, and her refraction was verified. Again, she was able to read the center of a line, but missed the letters on the right or the left of each line. She had bifocal lenses and was able to read 12 point type with the right eye and 8 point type with the left eye, through the center of her lenses (not the bifocals). Using a gooseneck lamp for illumination, she was able to read 4 point type using both eyes.

Her mimeographed homework assignments were printed in light purple. Contrast was greatly increased by placing the mimeographed sheet within a yellow acetate folder; with this simple adaptation she was able to read the assignment much more easily.

Because of her limited central visual field, Deidre has difficulty with crossword puzzle-type assignments and adding columns of numbers. I explained why she was having this problem to Deidre and her parents. She was much more successful when she used a dark card as a template to the side of a column of numbers to be added or to underline text to be read. She was also encouraged to remove her glasses and hold items closer if she has difficulty reading them.

In addition, a letter was written to her school principal describing Deidre's visual status and how it would affect her school work (see Illustration 1).

Susan Becker:

In providing services to a child or adolescent, there are three areas to consider: the child, the family, and school/educational issues. School is the second most important aspect of a child's life. It is his or her job and social milieu, and educational experiences shape future vocational potential. It is important to look at the differences between a child's behavior in school and at home. Parents must learn what the child's needs are in school, and school personnel must understand the needs that the child brings from home.

Illustration 1

HAMMOND MEDICAL CENTER
Hammond, IN 44444

Mr. John A. Smith, Principal
Hammond Elementary School
123 Main Street
Hammond, IN 44444

Dear Mr. Smith:

I performed a complete ophthalmological examination on Deidre Edwards on 10/9/90, with a follow-up exam on 10/19/90.

Her best corrected vision (with glasses) varies from 20/50 to 20/70. Her vision is impaired, but it is functional for most tasks. She has a restricted central visual field. It is likely that her vision will vary at times and may become worse in either eye, but she will retain functional vision.

She should be expected to participate fully in all school activities and should not be permitted to use her visual impairment as an excuse for not doing well in her school work.

Several adaptations in her classroom will be helpful:

• Deidre has difficulty reading print in normal classroom lighting; however, using a gooseneck light, she can read telephone book size print. She will need to sit near an electrical outlet in order to use the lamp.

• She needs to use a bold pen to do her homework assignments, tests, and other routine school work.

• She needs to hold the material she is reading close to her eyes, perhaps removing her glasses to read. Please reassure her teachers that this will not hurt her or strain her eyes.

• Using a template, a contrasting sheet of colored paper, or a dark ruler to underline what she is reading will be very helpful, especially with math problems or crossword puzzle exercises. Placing a yellow acetate sheet over mimeographed assignments will provide better contrast and will make them easier for her to read.

If you have any questions, please call me at 333-1111. Again, Deidre should be expected to do all work normally and perform well.

Sincerely,

Alice G. Karpik, MD

cc: Mr. and Mrs. Edwards

A basic social work assessment should be done in order to understand who Deidre is, who her family is, and how they may react to vision loss; to suggest interventions; and to explain why certain recommendations may or may not work.

Some of the questions that should be asked are:

• How is Deidre reacting to this vision loss? What issues is she grappling with and how does loss of vision affect those issues?

• Does Deidre have good friends? How are they reacting to her vision loss? Do they even know about it?

• What kind of social supports does this family have? Do close relatives live nearby? Does Deidre belong to any groups? Does her family attend church or synagogue?

• What age were her parents when they had cataracts? Are they comfortable talking about their own experiences?

• How does the family as a whole view Deidre's vision loss? How do they view their own visual impairments?

• Do Mom and Dad show up for appointments, or just Mom? Who is handling this "crisis?"

• Are there siblings who have experienced similar visual difficulties?

• What did the optometrist tell the family when he or she measured an acuity of 20/200 in Deidre's right eye?

• Does Deidre wear her glasses regularly at school and at home? Is fatigue a factor for her when she is doing her school work?

The ophthalmologist should recommend that a functional vision evaluation be made by a teacher of the visually impaired to check that all possible accommodations have been made in the classroom and to discuss with the classroom teacher other possible changes that might help Deidre function to the best of her ability. Simple interventions such as allowing additional time for taking tests can help a student with a visual impairment to succeed rather than become frustrated and fail.

How difficult is it for Deidre to read from the blackboard? Should the classroom teacher state verbally what she has put on the board? A look at Deidre's reading skills will help our understanding of how her vision loss is affecting her school work. What reading group is she in? How are her fine motor skills? If her handwriting is illegible or if it takes her a very long time to complete an assignment, typing lessons might be recommended. Typing is also a very useful skill in the event that there is further loss of vision and extremely useful when learning computer skills. A consultation with the physical education teacher will alert him or her to Deidre's limitations and provide an opportunity to discuss how modifications may be made so that she can participate in games and sports. After the functional vision evaluation, recommendations will be made for services, which may be on a consultation basis or may involve weekly or daily modification of classroom materials.

The teacher of the visually impaired needs to inform the eye care professional about any fatigue or difficulty that Deidre experiences during the school day, changes in mood, or withdrawal that may indicate vision changes. The teacher should tell the eye care professional what specific services are being provided by the school system so that he or she understands the patient's needs. Since the medical profession is so highly respected, the eye care professional is often the key to ensuring school compliance with education plan recommendations. Letters from eye care professionals can be used effectively to reinforce student independence, ensuring that a student is allowed to participate in school activities but limiting any activities that place the student in danger.

There are many good suggestions given in the letter from the ophthalmologist to the principal and they are reasonably stated. A copy of the letter should be sent to the classroom teacher. Many times information from the student's file never finds its way to the classroom teacher.

The family needs to be assured that there is information and assistance available and that they can accept as much or as little help as they choose. Deidre and her family need to learn advocacy skills so that they can make their needs known to educational, medical, and rehabilitation personnel. They need to learn what their rights are in terms of special education meetings and individual education plans (IEP). There are local and national parents' groups and advocacy organizations that can educate and assist parents, but the real training often comes when the teacher accompanies parents to their first educational plan meeting. Local politics, budgetary restrictions, and the "way we've always done it" all make each meeting unique and challenging.

Strong collaboration between the teacher of the visually impaired and the eye care professional is important to ensure that the whole child is considered when making educational plans and helping parents follow through at home.

Elsie Dunbar: An Older Woman with Vision and Hearing Losses

John Mascia, M.A., Audiologist
Martha Bagley, M.S., Specialist to Older Adults

<u>Assessment</u>:   Hearing: gradual moderate-severe sensorineural hearing loss, bilaterally, commencing 8 years ago (as reported by client). Vision: moderate (LE) to severe (RE) loss of visual field due to chronic undetected glaucoma. Early cataracts, more advanced in the left eye. Acuity 20/100 (R.E.) and 20/70 (L.E.).

Until three years ago, Elsie Dunbar, a 76 year old widowed grandmother of four, was president of her church's senior activity group. She loved needlework and founded the quilting group at a local senior center. She and several close friends regularly met for lunch at a popular local cafe. Mrs. Dunbar felt especially fortunate to have a large family. Her son, who lives out of state, called every Sunday afternoon, an event that Mrs. Dunbar always looked forward to.

Over the last three years, Mrs. Dunbar has gradually isolated herself from her friends and family. Her inappropriate responses to questions led her family and friends to wonder if she was becoming senile. Her sense of direction was not what it used to be. Mrs. Dunbar dropped out of her church and the senior center activities. She has not been to a restaurant or completed any needlework in several years.

Although the family knew that she did not hear or see as well as she once did, the extent of the problem did not become clear until Mrs. Dunbar did not answer the telephone one Sunday afternoon. Her son called his mother's neighbor in a panic and asked if she would check the house. Mrs. Dunbar was fine; she just did not hear the phone. Obvious-

Susan L. Greenblatt, (ed.) Meeting the Needs of People with Vision Loss: A Multidisciplinary Perspective,   Lexington, MA: Resources for Rehabilitation

ly, Mrs. Dunbar's sensory losses appeared to be more serious than originally suspected.

At the insistence of her son, Mrs. Dunbar visited an audiologist recommended by her family doctor and received a hearing test. The audiologist found a moderate to severe hearing loss with depressed speech discrimination abilities. He told Mrs. Dunbar that she was a candidate for a hearing aid; however, given the depressed speech discrimination abilities, even with a hearing aid she still would not hear every word. The audiologist told her that she would need to speechread (lipread) also. Mrs. Dunbar was reluctant to get a hearing aid and felt that speechreading would be too difficult given her vision difficulties. The audiologist also encouraged her to get an eye examination.

Mrs. Dunbar visited an ophthalmologist recommended by her family doctor. The examination revealed loss in the visual field from glaucoma, cataracts in the early stages of development, and reduced visual acuity. The ophthalmologist prescribed medications to control the glaucoma and bifocal glasses to accommodate for presbyopia and assist her with reading, and also referred her to a low vision specialist.

The low vision specialist discussed with Mrs. Dunbar a number of techniques for better utilizing her reduced visual field, such as scanning, localization, and spotting. She also recommended some strategies that Mrs. Dunbar could use to perform reading and sewing tasks, such as increasing lighting and working on contrasting backgrounds, and loaned her several magnifiers.

Mrs. Dunbar finally ordered hearing aids from the audiologist and reported an improvement in her hearing. She still had difficulty understanding speech, especially in noisy conditions. The audiologist again counseled her regarding speechreading. As much as Mrs. Dunbar might try, speech reading always seemed too difficult. People always spoke too fast, sat in the wrong place, turned their heads away, mumbled, or became irritated if she tried to get close enough to "really" see.

The audiologist also introduced Mrs. Dunbar to a number of assistive listening devices. An assistive listening device screens out background noise while amplifying only those sounds of interest, usually

124

speech. This is accomplished through placement of the microphone close to the sounds of interest. In contrast, a hearing aid amplifies all environmental sounds equally. Mrs. Dunbar tried a variety of devices including an FM (radio) system, an infrared system, an induction loop, and a hardwired system. She chose the system that best fits her needs in terms of cost, flexibility, and ease of operation.

Mrs. Dunbar's family purchased her assistive listening system. Although Medicaid covers hearing aids, it does not provide for assistive listening devices. Her hearing test could have been covered under Medicare; however, she utilized her private insurance.

Mrs. Dunbar's situation seemed to stabilize. She began doing some needlework again and visiting with friends. She even used her assistive listening device when dining out with her friends. Unfortunately, she never finished any needlework; church and senior center groups never became manageable; and her family continued to worry about her.

Mrs. Dunbar continued to have regular eye examinations. Eventually the ophthalmologist recommended cataract surgery. Mrs. Dunbar experienced improvement in her vision following the surgery, and she began to get out more and finish some needlework. Mrs. Dunbar also noticed what she thought was an increase in hearing. The audiologist also noticed an improvement in Mrs. Dunbar's communication abilities; however, upon testing, no change in the audiogram was noted. It suddenly became clear to Mrs. Dunbar that her hearing had stayed the same, but because her vision had improved, she was able to pick up more environmental information, even speechreading a little.

Mrs. Dunbar began to re-acquaint herself with friends and family. She enjoyed using her amplified telephone and used her assistive listening device to attend lectures.

The audiologist referred her to a support group for people with hearing problems, where she learned strategies for coping with her hearing loss and communicating more effectively with friends and family. Through the low vision specialist, she learned about a special activity program at the senior center for people with vision problems. She now visits the ophthalmologist and audiologist regularly.

Jessica Lane:
A Child with De Morsier's Syndrome

Lawrence S. Evans, Ph.D., M.D., Ophthalmologist
Michael Bina, Ed.D., Special Educator

Lawrence S. Evans:

Jessica Lane is a 7 year old girl with de Morsier's syndrome, which was diagnosed when she was several months old. De Morsier's syndrome (also called septo-optic dysplasia) is a congenital malformation of the brain and optic nerve. A primary symptom of de Morsier's syndrome is hypoplasia, an underdevelopment of the optic nerve, which leads to variable poor vision. Jessica also had nystagmus (involuntary rapid, oscillatory movements of the eye), typical in individuals who have had early visual deprivation. De Morsier's syndrome is often accompanied by delayed development due to poor functioning of the pituitary gland, leading to hypothyroidism. Jessica's growth and thyroid hormone levels are normal.

When she came to the Loyola Low Vision Service, Jessica's visual acuity was 20/200 in her good eye without correction; she had no light perception in the other eye. The prescription in the glasses she brought with her corrected her acuity to 20/100 and reduced her astigmatism. With refraction, I was able to further correct her acuity to 20/80. Although this may seem to be an insignificant correction, I think that any improvement in visual acuity is important, especially in the case of functional vision in only one eye. I added one diopter of astigmatism to a spherical correction. With a 2.5X power clip-on telescope, her distance acuity became 20/50. For near vision, I dispensed a reading cap (a lens which fits on the telescope for close focus). The reading cap is necessary because of the difficulty in accommodating through a telescope. I also dispensed a 3X stand loupe and a 20 diopter hand-held magnifier. She

Susan L. Greenblatt, (ed.) Meeting the Needs of People with Vision Loss: A Multidisciplinary Perspective, Lexington, MA: Resources for Rehabilitation

127

was able to read Jaeger 5 print (1M) with either of these devices. Since she reported that the yellow filter I had tried during the refraction made her more comfortable, I prescribed a yellow tint for her glasses.

Jessica uses a headband to hold the glasses on her face comfortably. Otherwise, with the telescope clipped to her glasses and the reading cap on the telescope, she would have had to tip her head to balance her reading system.

Jessica does not use the telescope all the time. She has preferential seating in the classroom in order to be close to the chalkboard. She can read the print in textbooks for her current grade level but will need to use low vision aids to read the smaller print that is common in more advanced grade levels. In general, I believe that it is a good idea to prescribe the minimal number of aids to meet the patient's needs, but in this case the prescription of magnifiers will help her with reading as she continues her education. Since she will need low vision aids all of her life, why not give her an early start?

Michael Bina:

Dr. Evans spent a great deal of time with Jessica and her family and dispensed a variety of low vision aids appropriate for different situations. He knew how she was functioning in school, which is very important. I am very pleased with his efforts in this regard.

Many ophthalmologists are surprised to learn how school districts can help them with their patients. For example, I asked Dr. Evans about Jessica's visual fields and he said he really had difficulty obtaining accurate visual field measurements with such a young child. I told him that teachers of the visually impaired and orientation and mobility instructors are trained to do functional vision evaluations. Had he made inquiries to the public school system, he would have obtained this information.

When I asked Dr. Evans who had trained Jessica in the use of the aids, he responded that he did. He said she was very bright and picked up the skills quickly. I asked him if he had had another young patient who was not as bright or as quick a learner, who would do the training then? Dr. Evans said in that instance, he would have the patient come back to his office. This is commendable, but ophthalmologists should ask the school to assist them with this training. This would make it easier for the student to learn how to use and integrate the device into the home and school settings.

I would encourage ophthalmologists to indicate that the student needs low vision aids training on the medical report that goes to the school district. School districts normally provide training with low vision aids in different functional situations.

The report submitted by Dr. Evans had many commendable features. I was particularly interested in the diagnosis. Many times I receive reports that state that a given student has optic atrophy. Optic atrophy is a generic diagnosis, and it really does not provide much information. The details of the diagnosis that were provided in this instance regarding growth and hormone levels were very valuable. I am also interested whenever a student has a medical condition and uses certain medications which may prevent or restrict participation in physical education or other activities.

One major issue that I encounter frequently is that students often resist using low vision aids. But if the students start using aids at an early age, they are less likely to resist them. Also, adapting to the use of aids at an early age may prevent rejection of them during the teenage years, when students feel a strong need to be like their peers. In this case, Jessica was adjusting to reading with an acuity of 20/80. When she reaches junior high or high school, not only will the size of print decrease, but she will also have longer reading assignments, and the curriculum materials will become more abstract. Providing the best possible refraction and appropriate low vision aids at the earliest age can help boost her self confidence now and perhaps prevent problems in school later.

I think that the idea of a team working with a child is very important. I do not mean to imply that every time an aid is prescribed that a multidisciplinary team must be involved. However, neither ophthalmologists nor education or rehabilitation professionals should operate in isolation. Whenever they work together, the success of the person with low vision is significantly more likely.

I have not mentioned the parents and their role in this process. If the ophthalmologist, in isolation, prescribes the best device, and if he or she coordinates the training without planning for integration of the aid into the child's daily repertoire, success is unlikely. Parents and school professionals need to be an integral part of the process. If acceptance and integration of the device into the child's life are to become a reality, the parents must be knowledgeable, sensitive, and understanding about the many variables surrounding the child's visual condition. Some of this information concerns basic anatomy and pathology and their effects on normal visual functioning.

When an aid is prescribed, the parents must understand the effect the device has on functional vision, both positively and negatively. For example, an aid may improve central acuity, but it may reduce the size of the visual field. Parents, perhaps as much as the child, need "training" in the use of the device. A simulated experience introduces family members and others to the effects of the device; and how they might assist or interfere with their functioning. Parents are the best "teachers" in terms of encouraging the use of the aid in all activities. If a child uses the aid in school, but "gets by" without using it in recreational reading at home, acceptance of and reliance on the aid will probably never occur. However, if parents, the ophthalmologist, and education and rehabilitation professionals all encourage the child, then the probability of success is greatly enhanced. The ophthalmologist cannot work alone clinically and expect the child to accept and utilize any device; nor can the education or rehabilitation professional or the parents. All parties need to coordinate and pool their expertise, energies, and strategies.

The ophthalmologist plays a key role in working with parents and other professionals. Sending copies of all medical information and reports to the school is helpful. It is rather unlikely, given scheduling demands, that an ophthalmologist would participate in the annual meetings where the child's Individualized Education Plan (IEP) is developed. A detailed medical report which goes beyond the basic visual acuities and fields, diagnosis, and prognosis, addressed to the IEP committee is very helpful. In some cases, the ophthalmologist may

130

attend the committee meeting or participate via a telephone conference call.

Summing up, this case provides an example of exemplary assistance provided by the ophthalmologist. Not only did Dr. Evans focus on the medical situation, he also focused on Jessica's functional activities and strove to enable her to be successful in school, at home, and in the community.

Ophthalmologists will find that school staff can be very valuable in assisting them in the total comprehensive care of their patients. Keeping in touch with school staff and allowing them to sit in on the low vision evaluation will be beneficial to all parties concerned, especially to the patient for whom the ophthalmologist has responsibility.

Harold Faber: An Older Man with Stroke-Related Vision Loss

Stanley F. Wainapel, M.D., M.P.H., Physiatrist
Fran A. Weisse, L.C.S.W., Social Worker

Stanley F. Wainapel:

Harold Faber, an 89 year old recently retired engineer who was living independently in his apartment, was admitted to a hospital because of symptoms of visual loss and impaired ability to walk. Examination revealed an alert man with clear speech, mild right sided weakness, and a right visual field deficit. He was able to stand by himself but walked very hesitantly because of impaired balance and his right sided visual loss. CT scan of the brain revealed the presence of a fresh left occipital infarction. In subsequent days, he reported the appearance of imaginary human figures in his right visual field; he was aware that these were not real people but was nonetheless distressed by their presence.

A neuro-ophthalmology consult was obtained, and Mr. Faber was found to have a dense right homonymous hemianopsia with an otherwise normal ophthalmologic exam (clear lens, negative fundus exam, normal intraocular pressure, and extraocular movements). He was also diagnosed as having release hallucinations due to his acute vision loss.

He was evaluated by occupational and physical therapists while in the hospital. He could walk with a broad based gait without assistive devices but tended to bump into objects located on his right side. Since he was aware of his visual deficit, Mr. Faber was taught to look further than usual to his right in order to compensate for his hemianopsia. He declined to use a standard or quadruped cane and tended to think that he would manage adequately at home.

Susan L. Greenblatt, (ed.) Meeting the Needs of People with Vision Loss: A Multidisciplinary Perspective, Lexington, MA: Resources for Rehabilitation

However, after discharge from the hospital, he had great difficulty in conducting his activities of daily living (ADL), such as cooking, laundry, shopping, and with some personal care tasks such as shaving and grooming. An occupational therapist with special expertise in vision rehabilitation was consulted, and after assessing him, she also made several home visits to evaluate and teach him appropriate self-care techniques.

Mr. Faber was referred to a low vision clinic in a local facility which provides services to individuals who are blind or visually impaired. This referral was made with the expectation that magnifiers, reading guides, or special prism systems might help him to read, write, and perform other activities with greater success. He was also referred to the orientation and mobility program at the same facility to evaluate whether he might benefit from the use of a white cane as a means of increasing his outdoor mobility.

Fran A. Weisse:

Mr. Faber was very fortunate to have had a neuro-ophthalmology consult soon after hospital admission. Initial diagnostic examinations of stroke patients often fail to reveal visual deficits, such as visual neglect, when visual acuity is normal (Halligan et al.: 1991). (Visual neglect is the failure to compensate for the loss of visual field due to stroke.) Since Mr. Faber and his physician were aware of his right field deficits, he was taught to compensate by turning his head further to the right so that the object he was looking for would appear in his left visual fields.

It is unclear in this case presentation whether Mr. Faber received services in a rehabilitation setting or whether he was discharged directly from an acute care hospital. Participation in a stroke rehabilitation program might have detected his subsequent problems with activities of daily living and a more realistic understanding of his need to use a cane.

The occupational therapy services provided to Mr. Faber at home are very important, because older individuals often benefit most from home-based training with realistic short-term goals.

While I applaud the physician's referral to the low vision service for optical and/or nonoptical aids, it is important to note that factors such as motivation and overall health affect the successful prescription of such aids. Prisms are optical aids that are used to the change the area in the visual field where visual information is received. Fresnel prisms may be mounted on the lenses of eyeglasses so that items missing from the visual field may be seen. Mr. Faber may find that turning his head to find the object, a technique he learned in the hospital, achieves the same result without having to deal with compromised visual acuity (Faye: 1984). Many low vision practitioners use press-on, temporary, Fresnel lenses to determine the patient's tolerance before prescribing final lenses.

Mr. Faber may find that glasses with prisms are helpful in reading very important items, such as personal correspondence and bills, but he may prefer to use nonoptical aids for other daily activities. A typoscope or reading guide, made of black cardboard with a rectangular opening cut out of it, may help him read more comfortably by isolating several lines of type. He may wish to place his finger at the end of a column of print as a reference point as he reads back and forth from line to line.

For recreational reading, I would recommend the use of Talking Books to reduce stress and fatigue. These recorded books and magazines are available free-of-charge and are easy to use. Bold-line paper, bold pens, and a writing guide are good choices for correspondence and grocery lists; a cassette recorder is a useful alternative.

The referral for orientation and mobility services is an excellent idea. Orientation and mobility teachers not only provide instruction for outdoor cane travel but can also assess Mr. Faber's home, make suggestions for adaptations, and teach techniques to make him feel more comfortable moving around his apartment.

A rehabilitation teacher from the same local organization may offer services which supplement the occupational therapist's training. Rehabilitation teachers are very knowledgeable about the myriad adaptive aids available to help individuals with vision loss.

There is no mention of Mr. Faber's family in this case study. Family support is one of the most crucial aspects of recovery for stroke patients. Spouses and other family members should be included in meetings where the individual's rehabilitation programs are designed (Resources for Rehabilitation: 1990).

Mr. Faber may also benefit from participation in a stroke club, where members are stroke survivors and their families; a stroke support group, usually coordinated by a professional service provider; or a vision loss support group. In addition to practical information and emotional support, groups such as these often motivate the individual to seek out services such as day activity programs and respite care.

Mr. Faber's physician and rehabilitation team have made some excellent referrals, which will be enhanced with the services I have mentioned. All service providers should report Mr. Faber's progress to his rehabilitation team, noting his successes and their observations of any potential warning signs of another stroke, such as slurred speech and confusion.

References

Faye, Eleanor E.
1984   *Clinical Low Vision* Boston, MA: Little Brown and Co.

Halligan, Peter, B. Wilson, and J. Cockburn
1990   "A Short Screening Test for Visual Neglect in Stroke Patients" *International Disability Studies* 12:3:95-99

Resources for Rehabilitation
1990   *Resources for Elders with Disabilities* Lexington, MA: Resources for Rehabilitation

Living with Low Vision
A Resource Guide for People with Sight Loss

A LARGE PRINT (**18 point bold type**) comprehensive directory that helps people with sight loss locate the services, products, and publications that they need to keep reading, working, and enjoying life. Chapters for children, elders, and people with both hearing and vision loss plus information on self-help groups, how to keep working with vision loss, and making everyday living easier. Second edition. 1990
ISBN 0-929718-04-6 $35.00

Rehabilitation Resource Manual: VISION

A desk reference that enables professionals to make effective referrals. Includes information on understanding the responses to vision loss; breaking the news of irreversible vision loss; guidelines on starting self-help groups; information on professional research and service organizations; plus chapters on optical and nonoptical aids; for special populations; and by eye condition/disease. Third edition. 1990
ISBN 0-929718-05-4 $39.95

Providing Services for People with Vision Loss
A Multidisciplinary Perspective
Susan L. Greenblatt, Editor

Written by ophthalmologists, rehabilitation professionals, a physician who has experienced vision loss, and a sociologist, this book discusses how various professionals can work together to provide coordinated care for people with vision loss. Chapters include Vision Loss: A Patient's Perspective; Vision Loss: An Ophthalmologist's Perspective; Operating a Low Vision Aids Service; The Need for Coordinated Care; Making Referrals for Rehabilitation Services; Mental Health Services: The Missing Link; Self-Help Groups for People with Sight Loss; and Aids and Techniques that Help People with Vision Loss plus a Glossary. Also available on cassette. 1989 ISBN 0-929718-02-X $19.95

Meeting the Needs of People with Vision Loss
A Multidisciplinary Perspective
Susan L. Greenblatt, Editor

Written by rehabilitation professionals, physicians, and a sociologist, this book discusses how to provide appropriate information and how to serve special populations. Chapters include What People with Vision Loss Need to Know; Information and Referral Services for People with Vision Loss; The Role of the Family in the Adjustment to Blindness or Visual Impairment; Diabetes and Vision Loss: Special Considerations; Special Needs of Children and Adolescents; Older Adults with Vision and Hearing Losses; Providing Services to Visually Impaired Elders in Long Term Care Facilities; plus a series of Multidisciplinary Case Studies. Also available on cassette. 1991 ISBN 0-929718-07-0 $24.95

Resources for Elders with Disabilities

This **unique** resource directory provides information about the services and products that elders with disabilities need to function independently. Printed in **18 point bold** type, this book includes information on the diseases that cause common disabilities, the major rehabilitation networks, self-help groups, and legislation that affects people with disabilities. Chapters on hearing loss, vision loss, diabetes, arthritis, osteoporosis, and stroke describe assistive devices, organizations, and publications that help people with these conditions. 1990
ISBN 0-929718-03-8
$39.95

Resources for People with Disabilities
and Chronic Conditions

A comprehensive resource guide with chapters on spinal cord injury, low back pain, diabetes, multiple sclerosis, hearing and speech impairments, vision impairment and blindness, and epilepsy. Each chapter includes information about the disease or condition; psychological aspects of the condition; professional service providers; environmental adaptations; assistive devices; and descriptions of organizations, publications, and products. Chapters on rehabilitation services; laws that affect people with disabilities; and making everyday living easier. Special information for children is also included. 1991 ISBN 0-929718-06-2 $44.95

Meeting the Needs of Employees with Disabilities

A comprehensive resource guide that provides employers and counselors with the information they need to help people with disabilities retain or obtain employment. Includes information on government programs and laws, supported employment, training programs, environmental adaptations, and the needs of special population groups, such as people with chronic illness and students in transition from school to work. Chapters on mobility, vision, and hearing and speech impairments include information on organizations, adaptive equipment, and services that enable employers to accommodate the needs of employees with disabilities. 1991

ISBN 0-929718-08-9 $42.95

LARGE PRINT Publications Designed for Distribution by Professionals to People with Disabilities

Distributed by physicians and other health care professionals, rehabilitation professionals, social service agencies, and libraries, these publications serve as self-help guides for people with disabilities and chronic conditions. They include information on each condition, rehabilitation services and professionals, products, and resources that help people with disabilities and chronic conditions to live independently. Titles include *Living with Low Vision, How to Keep Reading with Vision Loss, Living with Age-Related Macular Degeneration, Living with Diabetic Retinopathy, Aids for Everyday Living with Vision Loss, Living with Hearing Loss, Living with Arthritis, After a Stroke,* and *Living with Diabetes.* **18 point bold type,** printed on ivory paper with black ink for maximum contrast. 8 1/2" by 11" Sold in minimum quantities of 25 copies per title. Write or call for complete list of titles and prices.

Shipping & handling: $25.00 or less, add $3.00; $25.01 to 50.00, add $5.00; $50.01 to 100.00, add $7.00; add $2.00 for each additional $100.00 or fraction of $100.00. For shipping to Canada, add $2.00 to shipping and handling charges. Foreign orders must be prepaid in US currency; please write for shipping charges.